Interventional Spine Procedures

Editor

CARLOS E. RIVERA

PHYSICAL MEDICINE AND REHABILITATION CLINICS OF NORTH AMERICA

www.pmr.theclinics.com

Consulting Editor
SANTOS F. MARTINEZ

February 2018 • Volume 29 • Number 1

ELSEVIER

1600 John F. Kennedy Boulevard • Suite 1800 • Philadelphia, Pennsylvania, 19103-2899

http://www.theclinics.com

PHYSICAL MEDICINE AND REHABILITATION CLINICS OF NORTH AMERICA Volume 29, Number 1
February 2018 ISSN 1047-9651, ISBN 978-0-323-57000-8

Editor: Lauren Boyle
Developmental Editor: Meredith Madeira

Reprints. For copies of 100 or more of articles in this publication, please contact the Commercial Reprints Department, Elsevier Inc., 360 Park Avenue South, New York, NY 10010-1710. Tel.: 212-633-3874; Fax: 212-633-3820; E-mail: reprints@elsevier.com.

Physical Medicine and Rehabilitation Clinics of North America (ISSN 1047-9651) is published quarterly by Elsevier Inc., 360 Park Avenue South, New York, NY 10010-1710. Months of issue are February, May, August, and November. Business and Editorial Offices: 1600 John F. Kennedy Blvd., Suite 1800, Philadelphia, PA 19103-2899. Customer Service Office: 3251 Riverport Lane, Maryland Heights, MO 63043. Periodicals postage paid at New York, NY and additional mailing offices. Subscription price per year is $294.00 (US individuals), $571.00 (US institutions), $100.00 (US students), $351.00 (Canadian individuals), $752.00 (Canadian institutions), $210.00 (Canadian students), $427.00 (foreign individuals), $752.00 (foreign institutions), and $210.00 (foreign students). Foreign air speed delivery is included in all *Clinics* subscription prices. All prices are subject to change without notice. **POSTMASTER:** Send address changes to *Physical Medicine and Rehabilitation Clinics of North America*, Customer Service Office: Elsevier Health Sciences Division, Subscription Customer Service, 3251 Riverport Lane, Maryland Heights, MO 63043. **Customer Service: 1-800-654-2452 (US). From outside of the United States, call 314-447-8871. Fax: 314-447-8029. E-mail: JournalsCustomer Service-usa@elsevier.com (for print support); JournalsOnlineSupport-usa@elsevier.com (for online support).**

Physical Medicine and Rehabilitation Clinics of North America is indexed in *Excerpta Medica, MEDLINE/ PubMed (Index Medicus), Cinahl,* and *Cumulative Index to Nursing and Allied Health Literature.*

Contributors

CONSULTING EDITOR

SANTOS F. MARTINEZ, MD, MS
Diplomate of the American Academy of Physical Medicine and Rehabilitation, Certificate of Added Qualification Sports Medicine, Assistant Professor, Department of Orthopaedics, Campbell Clinic Orthopaedics, The University of Tennessee, Memphis, Tennessee, USA

EDITOR

CARLOS E. RIVERA, MD
Staff Physician, Campbell Clinic Orthopaedics, Memphis, Tennessee, USA

AUTHORS

JESSICA ARIAS GARAU, MD, FAAPMR
Interventional Pain Management Physician, Advanced Orthopedics and Sports Medicine Institute, Freehold, New Jersey, USA

DAVID ATKINS-GONZÁLEZ, MD
Resident Physician, Rehabilitation Medicine Service, VA Caribbean Healthcare System, San Juan, Puerto Rico, USA

KEVIN BARRETTE, MD
Department of Orthopaedic Surgery, Physical Medicine and Rehabilitation, Stanford University, Redwood City, California, USA

CARLOS E. CALVO, MD
Staff Physician, Rehabilitation Medicine Service, VA Caribbean Healthcare System, San Juan, Puerto Rico, USA

KE-VIN CHANG, MD, PhD
Department of Physical Medicine and Rehabilitation, National Taiwan University Hospital, Bei-Hu Branch, National Taiwan University College of Medicine, Taipei, Taiwan

ALLEN S. CHEN, MD, MPH
Director of Physiatry for the New York Presbyterian/Columbia Spine Hospital, Assistant Professor, Department of Rehabilitation and Regenerative Medicine, Columbia University Medical Center, Harkness Pavillion, New York, New York, USA

MICHELLE CHI, MD
Chief Resident, Department of Rehabilitation and Regenerative Medicine, New York Presbyterian Hospital of Columbia and Cornell, Harkness Pavillion, New York, New York, USA

EDUARDO J. CRUZ, MD
Spine & Sports, Ocala Family Medical Center, Assistant Professor, Ocala Regional Medical Center, Ocala, Florida, USA

ANTHONY A. CUNEO, MD, PhD
Interventional Pain Management Physician, The Orthopedic Group, Pittsburgh, Pennsylvania, USA

BRADLEY D. FULLERTON, MD
Private Practice, ProloAustin, Austin, Texas, USA; Clinical Assistant Professor, Department of Internal Medicine, Texas A&M College of Medicine, Bryan, Texas, USA

MICHAEL B. FURMAN, MD, MS
Fellowship Director, Interventional Spine and Sports, OSS Health, York, Pennsylvania, USA; Special Consultant, Rehabilitation Medicine, Sinai Hospital, Baltimore, Maryland, USA; Clinical Assistant Professor, Physical Medicine and Rehabilitation, Temple University, Lewis Katz School of Medicine, Philadelphia, Pennsylvania, USA

EDA GÜRÇAY, MD
Associate Professor, Department of Physical and Rehabilitation Medicine, Gaziler Training and Research Hospital, Ankara, Turkey

LIZA HERNÁNDEZ-GONZÁLEZ, MD
Staff Physician, Rehabilitation Medicine Service, VA Caribbean Healthcare System, San Juan, Puerto Rico, USA

LAWRENCE McLEAN HOUSE, MD
Department of Anesthesia and Perioperative Care, University of California San Francisco, San Francisco, California, USA

MURAT KARA, MD
Associate Professor, Department of Physical and Rehabilitation Medicine, Hacettepe University Faculty of Medicine, Ankara, Turkey

BAYRAM KAYMAK, MD
Professor, Department of Physical and Rehabilitation Medicine, Hacettepe University Faculty of Medicine, Ankara, Turkey

RYAN MATTIE, MD
Department of Anesthesiology, University of California San Francisco, San Francisco, California, USA

SIMONE MAYBIN, MD
Department of Physical Medicine and Rehabilitation, Vanderbilt University Medical Center, Nashville, Tennessee, USA

ZACHARY L. McCORMICK, MD
Division of Physical Medicine and Rehabilitation, The University of Utah, Salt Lake City, Utah, USA

EDUARDO OTERO LOPERENA, MD
Resident, Physical Medicine and Rehabilitation Residency Program, VA Caribbean Healthcare System, San Juan, Puerto Rico, USA

LEVENT ÖZÇAKAR, MD
Professor, Department of Physical and Rehabilitation Medicine, Hacettepe University
Faculty of Medicine, Ankara, Turkey

CARLOS E. RIVERA, MD
Staff Physician, Campbell Clinic Orthopaedics, Memphis, Tennessee, USA

BYRON J. SCHNEIDER, MD
Assistant Professor, Department of Physical Medicine and Rehabilitation, Vanderbilt
University Medical Center, Nashville, Tennessee, USA

DAVID A. SOTO QUIJANO, MD, FAAPMR
Director, Physical Medicine and Rehabilitation Residency Program, VA Caribbean
Healthcare System, San Juan, Puerto Rico, USA

ERIC STUROS, MD
Department of Physical Medicine and Rehabilitation, Vanderbilt University Medical
Center, Nashville, Tennessee, USA

BRADY WAHLBERG, DO
Interventional Spine and Sports Medicine, OSS Health, York, Pennsylvania, USA

WEI-TING WU, MD
Department of Physical Medicine and Rehabilitation, National Taiwan University Hospital,
Bei-Hu Branch, National Taiwan University College of Medicine, Taipei, Taiwan

Contents

Foreword   xiii

Santos F. Martinez

Preface   xv

Carlos E. Rivera

Cervical Epidural Steroid Injection: Techniques and Evidence   1

Lawrence McLean House, Kevin Barrette, Ryan Mattie, and Zachary L. McCormick

Cervical epidural steroid injections are a common treatment of cervical radicular pain. Important safety considerations include attention to the possibility of spinal cord infarction and spinal epidural hematoma. When appropriate, radiographic, technical, and pharmacologic principals are used, these procedures are relatively safe. Cervical epidural steroid injections are effective for the short-term treatment of radicular pain. More rigorously designed clinical outcomes studies of both cervical interlaminar and transforaminal epidural steroid injections are needed.

Image and Contrast Flow Pattern Interpretation for Attempted Epidural Steroid Injections   19

Michael B. Furman and Anthony A. Cuneo

Fluoroscopically guided, contrast-enhanced epidural steroid injections (ESIs) are frequently performed for radicular symptoms. Interventionalists performing these procedures should have a thorough and detailed understanding of spinal anatomy to safely and effectively deliver the desired injectate to the targeted site. Being able to differentiate epidural from nonepidural contrast flow is vital as is recognizing flow to undesired locations. This article summarizes the characteristics that distinguish between ideal epidural flow patterns and nonideal subarachnoid, intradural, and other suboptimal contrast flow patterns. Recognizing these patterns is essential for safe and successful ESIs and to prevent avoidable complications.

Lumbosacral Transitional Segments: An Interventional Spine Specialist's Practical Approach   35

Michael B. Furman, Brady Wahlberg, and Eduardo J. Cruz

The presence of a lumbosacral transitional vertebrae (LSTV) should prompt a more detailed preprocedural evaluation of the vertebral column to accurately determine spinal levels. An LSTV should prompt the use of corroborating intraprocedural imaging to verify morphology. The most important factors in treating lumbosacral transitional segments are communication among treating physicians to ensure segmental enumeration consistency and associated appropriate patient treatment.

Ultrasound for Lumbar Spinal Procedures   49

Michelle Chi and Allen S. Chen

> Ultrasonography has become an increasingly valuable and promising tool
> for performing image-guided spine interventions. The increase in the use
> of ultrasound has led to more studies evaluating ultrasound-guided inter-
> ventional spine procedures in comparison with fluoroscopy and computed
> tomography. Several studies have investigated the use of ultrasound for
> lumbosacral pain management procedures with favorable outcomes.

Peripheral Nerve Radiofrequency Neurotomy: Hip and Knee Joints   61

Liza Hernández-González, Carlos E. Calvo, and David Atkins-González

> Intraarticular hip and knee pain is a common cause of physical and psy-
> chosocial disability. Many conservative treatment options provide only
> short-term relief. Recent research has shown improvement in pain and
> function with minimal complications after radiofrequency neurotomy of
> the hip and the knee, especially in patients who have failed conservative
> treatment or are not surgical candidates. More quality research is needed
> to establish the efficacy and safety of these procedures in patients with re-
> fractory hip and knee pain.

Lumbar Epidural Steroid Injections   73

Carlos E. Rivera

> Lumbar epidural steroid injections under fluoroscopic guidance are used
> very commonly for the treatment of low back and lower extremity radicular
> pain. These procedures have been shown to be effective for pain relief in
> the short term and are relatively safe. The indications, evidence, and safety
> considerations for 2 different techniques, namely, interlaminar and trans-
> foraminal, are discussed.

Ultrasound-Guided Interventions of the Cervical Spine and Nerves   93

Ke-Vin Chang, Wei-Ting Wu, and Levent Özçakar

> High-resolution ultrasound (US) imaging enables prompt depiction of mus-
> cles, tendons, ligaments, and peripheral nerves. It seems to be the best
> imaging modality for guiding perineural injections. The most complicated
> neurovascular network of the musculoskeletal system surrounds the cer-
> vical spine, so injection to that region is never an easy task. This article
> elaborates the regional anatomy and the use of US scanning and guidance
> for cervical interventions, for example, cervical root, superficial cervical
> plexus, stellate ganglion, cervical medial branch, greater occipital nerve,
> and third occipital nerve. The article aims to lead readers to practice
> US-guided cervical injections precisely and safely.

**Sonographic Guide for Botulinum Toxin Injections of the Neck Muscles in Cervical
Dystonia**   105

Bayram Kaymak, Murat Kara, Eda Gürçay, and Levent Özçakar

> Intramuscular botulinum toxin (BoTX) injection is the first-line treatment
> of cervical dystonia. Poor treatment outcomes and some side effects,

however, have been reported after BoTX applications. One of the most important reasons is incorrect localization of the needle during toxin injections. Without imaging, it is impossible to verify precise needle positioning in the proper muscle. Ultrasound imaging has been recommended because of its high capability in illustrating most of the neck muscles. This article discusses how ultrasound imaging can be used to scan/access neck muscles, mainly from the perspective of BoTX injections.

Prolotherapy for the Thoracolumbar Myofascial System   125

Bradley D. Fullerton

 Video content accompanies this article at http://www.pmr.theclinics. com.

Prolotherapy has focused on entheses as a key source of chronic low back pain, even without clear diagnosis of enthesopathy. Treatment has traditionally been guided by anatomic knowledge and careful palpation. This article integrates ultrasonographic diagnosis of fascial injury with examination findings taught in traditional prolotherapy technique. Thoracolumbar fascial anatomy and biotensegrity theory are used to explain patient presentation and response to treatment at these pathologic findings. Detailed case reports provide proof of concept for the 60-year history of prolotherapy in the treatment of chronic low back pain.

Radiofrequency Denervation of the Cervical and Lumbar Spine   139

Jessica Arias Garau

Facet or zygapophysial joint pain is commonly seen in the aging population. Interventional procedures, such as facet joint nerve blocks, facet intraarticular injections, and radiofrequency denervation, are used for the diagnosis and treatment of axial spinal chronic neck and low back pain. The focus of this article is to understand how radiofrequency denervation works in the cervical and lumbar spine and to be able to properly select appropriate patients who might benefit from this safe and effective procedure.

Safety and Complications of Cervical Epidural Steroid Injections   155

Byron J. Schneider, Simone Maybin, and Eric Sturos

Serious neurologic complications following cervical transforaminal epidural steroid injections (CTFESI) and cervical interlaminar epidural steroid injections (CILESI) have been reported. For CILESI, this is caused by aberrant needle placement or space-occupying lesions, such as hematoma or abscess. For CTFESI, this is caused by embolic infarct when inadvertent intraarterial injection of particulate steroids has occurred. Multiple safety techniques are used to mitigate the risk of these serious complications. The most common adverse events that occur following CTFESI or CILESI are procedural-related pain, steroid side effects, and vasovagal reactions, which are relatively minor and self-limited.

Sacroiliac Joint Interventions   171

David A. Soto Quijano and Eduardo Otero Loperena

Sacroiliac joint (SIJ) pain is an important cause of lower back problems. Multiple SIJ injection techniques have been proposed over the years to help in the diagnosis and treatment of this condition. However, the SIJ innervation is complex and variable, and truly intraarticular injections are sometimes difficult to obtain. Different sacroiliac joint injections have been shown to provide pain relief in patients with this ailment. Various techniques for intraarticular injections, sacral branch blocks and radiofrequency ablation, both fluoroscopy guided and ultrasound guided, are discussed in this article. Less common techniques, such as prolotherapy, platelet-rich plasma injections, and botulism toxin injections, are also discussed.

PHYSICAL MEDICINE AND REHABILITATION CLINICS OF NORTH AMERICA

FORTHCOMING ISSUES

May 2018
Para Sports Medicine
Yetsa A. Tuakli-Wosornu and
Wayne Derman, *Editors*

August 2018
**Muscle Over-activity in Upper Motor Neuron
Syndrome: Assessment and Problem Solving
for Complex Cases**
Miriam Segal, *Editor*

November 2018
Value-Added Electrodiagnostics
Karen Barr and Ileana M. Howard, *Editors*

RECENT ISSUES

November 2017
**Promoting Health and Wellness in the
Geriatric Patient**
David A. Soto-Quijano, *Editor*

August 2017
Pelvic Pain
Kelly M. Scott, *Editor*

May 2017
Traumatic Brain Injury Rehabilitation
Blessen C. Eapen and David X. Cifu, *Editors*

RELATED INTEREST

Clinics in Sports Medicine, October 2016 (Vol. 35, Issue 4)
Return to Play Following Musculoskeletal Injury
Brett D. Owens, *Editor*

VISIT THE CLINICS ONLINE!
Access your subscription at:
www.theclinics.com

Foreword

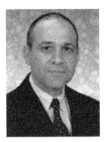

Santos F. Martinez, MD, MS
Consulting Editor

The Interventional Spine subspecialty has been a great success story within our field of Physical Medicine and Rehabilitation. It has also served as a catalyst for the evolvement of other peripheral interventional pursuits, such as musculoskeletal ultrasound. Dr Rivera presents a fine balance between academic and clinical descriptions of not only well-established interventional techniques but also evolving areas in this field. His presentation platform serves both the seasoned interventionalist and those in training who have an interest in incorporating procedure-based approaches in their clinical practice. Despite the clear descriptions of techniques, a formal apprenticeship or fellowship is still necessary for the interested practitioner before incorporating these techniques in their practice.

Indeed, we are at an interesting point in the interventional field as new technology will give the physiatrist more tools, equipment, and techniques to offer our patients. I thank and commend Dr Rivera and the authors for this great issue. Prior issues addressing regenerative and office-based ultrasound techniques may be of additional interest to the practitioner.

Santos F. Martinez, MD, MS
American Academy of Physical Medicine
and Rehabilitation
Campbell Clinic Orthopaedics
Department of Orthopaedics
University of Tennessee
Memphis, TN 38104, USA

E-mail address:
smartinez@campbellclinic.com

Phys Med Rehabil Clin N Am 29 (2018) xiii
https://doi.org/10.1016/j.pmr.2017.10.002
1047-9651/18/© 2017 Published by Elsevier Inc.

Preface

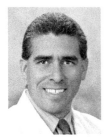

Carlos E. Rivera, MD
Editor

It is a great pleasure and honor to serve as Guest Editor of *Physical Medicine and Rehabilitations Clinics of North America* on Interventional Spine Procedures. Spinal problems are the most common musculoskeletal complaints we face and are very complex and multidimensional. Patients with spinal complaints are bread and butter in our day-to-day clinics. As rehabilitation specialists, we learn to try to address issues through a conservative approach, dealing with the patient as a whole entity, emphasizing the identification of functional deficits that can be treated or improved with exercise. Unfortunately, despite our best efforts with conservative, noninvasive protocols, many patients continue with limitations due to pain that affect their daily activities, causing a strain in their day-to-day activities, including work, home activities, exercise, social activities, and hobbies.

The objective of this issue is to provide an overview of different sources of chronic spinal pain, including both deep and more superficial soft tissue conditions and options for treating these problems with interventional procedures. We include reviews for procedures performed with fluoroscopic and/or ultrasound guidance, including epidural steroid injections to alleviate pain from deep structures like spinal nerves, radiofrequency denervation of the zygapophyseal joints, and also interventional procedures for soft tissues/myofascial deficits. The sacroiliac joint as well as the hip and knee is included as many patients with spinal issues also have problems in these areas, and addressing them as part of the treatment can be very effective and help resolve some chronic accompanying nonresponsive type of pains.

Interventional procedures are an excellent tool to have in our armamentarium for patients that because of pain can't progress through their rehabilitation program or in which the pain limits their day-to-day activities, affecting their quality of life. The reviews in this issue provide not only evidence of the indications and effectiveness of the procedures but also technical details that could help everyone, especially the more novice practitioners like our residents and fellows. Reviews on safety and complications as well as in abnormal contrast flow patterns on attempted epidural injections will also be included to keep with our goal of maintaining a "do no harm" approach.

Phys Med Rehabil Clin N Am 29 (2018) xv–xvi
http://dx.doi.org/10.1016/j.pmr.2017.08.013
1047-9651/18/© 2017 Published by Elsevier Inc.

pmr.theclinics.com

I hope you enjoy this issue. I really appreciate, and want to thank, all the contributing authors for their time and sharing their knowledge with all.

Carlos E. Rivera, MD
Campbell Clinic Orthopedics
8000 Centerview Parkway, Suite 500
Memphis, TN 38018, USA

E-mail address:
crivera@campbellclinic.com

Cervical Epidural Steroid Injection
Techniques and Evidence

Lawrence McLean House, MD[a], Kevin Barrette, MD[b],
Ryan Mattie, MD[c], Zachary L. McCormick, MD[d],*

KEYWORDS

- Injections • Epidural • Neck pain • Evidence-based medicine

KEY POINTS

- Cervical epidural steroid injections are a common interventional treatment of cervical radicular pain.
- The differing neurovascular anatomy in proximity to the route of entry for transforaminal and interlaminar epidural steroid injections must be thoroughly understood to perform safe injections.
- Use of particulate steroid and mixture with certain local anesthetics may pose increased risk for spinal cord ischemia during transforaminal epidural injection, in which inadvertent arterial injection is possible.
- Cervical epidural steroid injections are effective short-term treatment of radicular pain.
- The evidence base for cervical epidural steroid injections is limited by true placebo-controlled trials.

INTRODUCTION
Epidemiology

Neck pain is the fourth leading cause of disability in the United States. The lifetime risk of developing cervicalgia approaches 50% in the general population.[1,2] Cervical radiculopathy is a pathologic cause of neck pain, often accompanied by radiating upper extremity pain. Mechanical compression of cervical nerve roots, usually by age-related cervical spondylosis or disk herniation results in ischemic nerve damage.[3]

Disclosure Statement: The authors have nothing to disclose.
[a] Department of Anesthesia and Perioperative Care, University of California San Francisco, 513 Parnassus Avenue, 436, San Francisco, CA 94143, USA; [b] Department of Orthopaedic Surgery, Physical Medicine and Rehabilitation, Stanford University, 450 Broadway Street, M/C 6342, Redwood City, CA 94063, USA; [c] Department of Anesthesiology, University of California San Francisco, 521 Parnassus Avenue, San Francisco, CA 94143, USA; [d] Division of Physical Medicine and Rehabilitation, University of Utah, 30 N 1900 E, Rm 1C441, Salt Lake City, UT 84132, USA
* Corresponding author.
E-mail address: Zachary.mccormick@ucsf.edu

Phys Med Rehabil Clin N Am 29 (2018) 1–17
https://doi.org/10.1016/j.pmr.2017.08.001
1047-9651/18/© 2017 Elsevier Inc. All rights reserved.
pmr.theclinics.com

Furthermore, proinflammatory pathways initiated by neural ischemia perpetuate and aggravate regional pain.[4] Cervical radiculopathy may be self-limited, but persistent pain, weakness, or paresthesia often prompts therapy efforts.

Treatment modalities for cervical radiculopathy include oral analgesics and neuropathic pain medication, physical therapy, manipulation, local injection of medication, and surgical decompression. Epidural injection of corticosteroids and local anesthetics (LAs) achieves a high concentration of the treating agent within the epidural space to inhibit inflammation and reduce nociceptive afferent signaling. The 2 most common approaches to cervical epidural steroid injections (ESIs), transforaminal (TFESI) and interlaminar (IESI),[5] are reviewed. Other neck cervical needle approaches (trigger point injections, acupuncture, and so forth) are omitted.

Indications for Cervical Epidural Steroid Injection

Cervical radicular pain
Cervical radiculitis
Cervical radiculopathy

Utilization

Cervical radiculopathy affects approximately 1 in 1000 adults per year.[6,7] Over the past decade, the rate of cervicothoracic ESIs has doubled (119% increase) among Medicare enrollees in the United States.[8] State-to-state utilization of ESIs varies from 5 to 40 interventions per 1000 Medicare enrollees.[9] The growth of cervical ESIs has accompanied a shift in their predominant setting from hospital-based sites to ambulatory surgery centers and outpatient physician offices.

Currently, there is lack of consensus regarding the ideal technique for Cervical ESI that balances safety and efficacy. This review outlines the 2 Cervical ESI approaches and means of optimizing safety and summarizes the highest-quality evidence for the clinical effectiveness of Cervical ESI.

CERVICAL TRANSFORAMINAL EPIDURAL STEROID INJECTION
Anatomy

A thorough understanding of cervical anatomy with particular attention to neurovascular structures is essential for the safe performance of cervical TFESI. One anterior spinal artery and 2 posterior spinal arteries provide penetrating branches that supply the cervical spinal cord. These arteries arise from radicular and spinal medullary arteries, which originate from the ascending cervical, deep cervical, and vertebral arteries. The spinal and radicular medullary arteries traverse the cervical neuroforamina, where they nourish the exiting spinal nerve root, penetrate the dura, and then anastomose with the anterior and posterior spinal arteries.[10,11] The vertebral arteries additionally provide blood supply to the brainstem and posterior regions of the brain. They traverse cephalad between the transverse foramina of the C2-C6 vertebrae, anterior to the cervical facet joints, and typically anterior to the ventral ramus of the cervical nerve root. Anatomic variations of their course are described.[12]

Given the proximity to the neuroforamina in the cervical spine, the spinal, radicular medullary, and vertebral arteries are of primary concern when approaching the transforaminal epidural space (**Fig. 1**). One cadaveric dissection study found more than 22% of cervical neuroforamina contained an arterial vessel within 2 mm of the needle trajectory using a posterior foraminal approach.[13] Although vertebral artery penetration itself is unlikely, anatomic variants must be considered. Furthermore, the extent to which arterial branches contribute to spinal circulation can further influence the possibility of a serious adverse event.

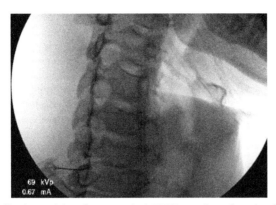

Fig. 1. Final needle tip position for a cervical TFESI, as viewed under fluoroscopy in an anterior-oblique plane. The needle tip resides a few millimeters anterior to the superior articular process in the posterior aspect of the right C6-C7 neuroforamen to avoid trespass of the vertebral artery and exiting nerve root.

Procedure Technique

Patient positioning for cervical TFESI is supine, oblique (swimmer's position), or lateral decubitus. The skin of the ipsilateral neck is cleaned with antibacterial solution and draped in sterile fashion. An anterior- posterior (AP) fluoroscopic view is obtained to identify bony anatomy relevant to the injection target. An oblique view is subsequently imaged to reveal best trajectory toward the aperture of the neuroforamen along its entire length, oriented in an anterolateral plane. The patient is cautioned not to move prior to needle insertion. The skin and superficial subcutaneous tissue are anesthetized using LA directly overlaying the posterior half of the targeted neuroforamen.

Then, a 25-gauge spinal needle is introduced. Using guidance from serial fluoroscopic images, the needle is advanced toward the anterior half of the superior articular process, at least 1 needle width posterior to the dorsal border of the neuroforamen. This touchpoint ideally restricts needle advancement posterior to the vertebral artery, any radiculomedullary arteries entering the neuro foramen, and the spinal nerve root. Contacting the periosteum of the superior articular process ensures that the needle is not advanced too far medially toward the thecal sac from the oblique view. The depth of insertion is evaluated in an AP view, with subsequent return to an oblique view. The needle is adjusted to pass tangential to the anterior surface of the superior articular process by a few millimeters (see **Fig. 1**). Returning to the AP view, the needle is advanced in small increments until the tip is opposite to the midline of the articular pillars. Restricting needle advancement posterior to the medial boundary line of the uncinate processes should ensure that the needle does not threaten puncturing the thecal sac. Once the needle has contacted this landmark, the tip is redirected into the posterior aspect of the neuroforamen at the midpoint of its craniocaudal diameter, and the medial depth of needle placement is confirmed in an AP fluoroscopic view.

As the needle is advanced into the neuroforamen, it may contact the spinal nerve or ventral ramus, which induces severe radicular pain or intense paresthesias. If this occurs, the needle should be withdrawn slightly. If sensations do not cease on withdrawal, the procedure should be discontinued. Sedation should be avoided or minimized during cervical TFESI, such that the patient is able to warn the clinician if such sensations are experienced. To confirm final needle tip placement, spot films are obtained in the oblique and AP views, again demonstrating needle position in the posterior aspect of the neuroforamen in the oblique view and the needle to be within the foramen but not medial to the uncinate line in the AP view. Aspiration should be attempted, although this is not a failproof safeguard against intravascular injection.[14] Under live fluoroscopy, a small volume of nonionic contrast medium is injected. Contrast spread pattern outlining the spinal nerve in the neuroforamen and entering the lateral epidural space suggests proper needle tip placement. Patients may report pain comparable to usual radicular symptoms. If this pain is tolerable, the injection may be continued. Assuming that contrast does not reveal aberrant placement into an artery, a vein, the subdural space, or the subarachnoid space, the steroid injectate can be safely deposited.[15]

Safety Considerations

Permanent neurologic complications arising from cervical TFESI are a serious concern; however, such events are rare. When ESIs are performed using current standards of care, permanent neurologic complications are even more rare.[16,17] Nonetheless, the cardinal complication of transforaminal cervical epidural injection is infarction of the central nervous system via inadvertent vascular injection,[11] and several safety considerations should be made prior to the procedure.

Particulate versus nonparticulate steroid use

The use of particulate (ie, triamcinolone, methylprednisolone, and betamethasone acetate) or nonparticulate steroid (ie, dexamethasone) represents an important safety consideration. Historically, particulate rather than nonparticulate steroids have been used for epidural injection due to assumed advantage associated with the depot effect the particulate agents. Multiple case reports, however, have demonstrated permanent neurologic compromise after cervical TFESI with a particulate agent.[18–20] Inadvertent intra-arterial (vertebral artery and radiculomedullary arteries) during cervical TFESI with particulate steroid may result in occlusion of the perfusing vasculature and subsequent in embolic infarction.

The mechanism for particulate steroid risk is supported by both in vivo and in vitro studies. Dexamethasone particles are 10-times smaller than red blood cells and do not aggregate under light microscopy. Particulate steroids, however, may contain particles larger than red blood cells and have been shown to aggregate.[21] An animal study demonstrated that direct vertebral artery injection of particulate steroids yield neurologic complications, whereas injection of nonparticulate steroids do not.[20] Furthermore, recent comparative clinic outcomes research suggests that no advantage exists for particulate versus nonparticulate corticosteroids with regard to pain reduction or functional outcomes.[22–28] Thus, a multidisciplinary pain workgroup recommends that nonparticulate steroids should be used exclusively when performing cervical TFESI.[11]

Local anesthetic use

An argument has been made that LA should not be used during cervical epidural injections due the possibility of inadvertent subdural or subarachnoid injection, which could lead to a high spinal block as well as inadvertent intra-arterial injection, which could lead to seizure.[22,29–31] Some providers continue to use LA in the epidural injectate. If this decision is elected, in addition to careful selection of steroid, the choice of anesthetic (should it be used) during cervical TFESI must also be considered. In a study by Hwang and colleagues,[32] combinations of 1 LA (ropivacaine, bupivacaine, and lidocaine) were mixed with 1 steroid solution (triamcinolone, dexamethasone, and betamethasone sodium phosphate) and observed under light microscopy while

NaOH was added and pH was recorded. Importantly, when mixed with dexamethasone, ropivacaine crystal precipitates larger than arterioles were observed at a physiologic pH (7.0). Alternatively, lidocaine and bupivacaine did not precipitate into crystals when mixed with dexamethasone. Although in vivo confirmation of these findings is needed, use of ropivacaine mixed with dexamethasone is not recommended during cervical TFESIs because embolization of a radiculomedulary artery with crystal precipitate is theoretically possible.

Digital subtraction technology

Given the risk of complications that can arise from intravascular injection of corticosteroids, an important tool for avoiding inadvertent intravascular injection is digital subtraction technology. Digital subtraction technology may be used in conjunction with live fluoroscopy. This technique involves an initial preinjection scout image or mask image (**Fig. 2**A) followed by injection of contrast agent under live observation (**Fig. 2**B and C). The pixel values from the original static image are subtracted from the image during contrast injection, which provides enhance visualization of contrast distribution because the relative intensity of all static structures is minimized.[33] Using the technology during cervical TFESI, detection of intravascular contrast flow is improved 1.5-fold to 2-fold compared with live fluoroscopy alone.[34] It must be emphasized that the theoretic increase in safety when using this digital subtraction technology assumes appropriate technique, including lack of patient movement (breathing, swallowing, and shifting), adequate volume of contrast injection, and recognition of a vascular contrast pattern by the clinician; this technology does not inherently prevent inadvertent vascular injection and subsequent adverse events.[35] Furthermore, digital subtraction technology during TFESI procedures has been shown to increase radiation exposure to patients 2-fold to 4-fold compared with conventional live fluoroscopy.[36] Thus, prudent rather than routine use of digital subtraction technology is currently recommended.[11]

CERVICAL INTERLAMINAR EPIDURAL STEROID INJECTION
Anatomy

A thorough understanding of cervical anatomy, unique to the dorsal epidural space and posterior elements, is crucial for safe cervical IESI. Significant differences in the vasculature and the width of the dorsal epidural space compared with the characteristics of these structures in the ventral epidural space result in alternative risks and considerations during cervical IESI as opposed to TFESI. First, unlike the neuroforaminal space, there is minimal to no arterial vasculature in the dorsal epidural space or the pathway from the skin to the goal final needle position. As a result, there is essentially no risk of ischemic neurologic infarction due to embolic phenomenon. A rich venous plexus in the dorsal epidural space leads, however, to a risk of epidural hematoma, which may result in spinal cord injury of compressive etiology. Permanent neurologic injury is of great concern in such cases, particularly if the hematoma is not decompressed rapidly; prognosis of neurologic recovery is improved if decompression is performed within 12 hours of symptom onset.[37]

The second major anatomy difference of the dorsal compared with the ventral cervical epidural space is AP dimension at ascending cranial levels. The dorsal epidural space is known to diminish at higher spinal levels; based on anatomic studies, the diameter shrinks rapidly above the C7-T1 level; it is approximately 1 mm to 2 mm in diameter at levels above C6-C7 and even less depending on individual variation, including the presence of spinal stenosis.[38] Thus, the risk of dural puncture or even direct spinal cord trauma increases significantly when the interlarminar epidural space is accessed above the C7-T1 level.

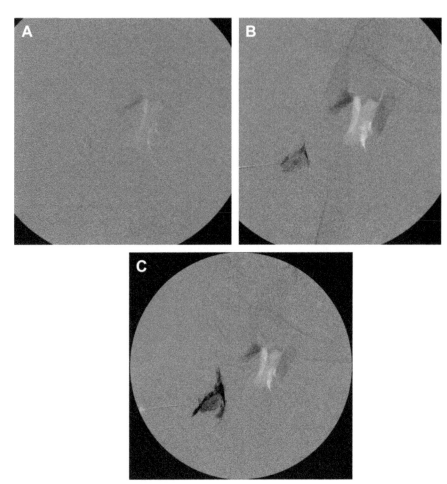

Fig 2. (A-C) Sequential images of a fluoroscopic digital subtraction study during a cervical TFESI procedure. (A) Digital subtraction mask image; these pixel values are subtracted from the subsequent images during live contrast injection to highlight distribution of the contrast agent. (B) Initial injection of contrast; the exiting nerve root is highlighted and cephalocaudal flow in the epidural space is apparent. (C) With the injection of additional contrast, it is apparent that contrast spreads along the exiting nerve root as well as to the adjacent cephalocaudal levels in the ipsilateral epidural space, without any apparent vascular, subdural, or subarachnoid uptake.

Procedure Technique

Given the anatomic considerations described previously, the goal of a cervical IESI is to place the tip of the needle minimally into the epidural space, sufficient for deposit of the injectate but without penetration of the dura. Landmark guidance is associated with an unacceptably high rate of inaccurate injections and safety concerns.[39] Clinical practice guidelines recommend that fluoroscopic guidance is used in all cervical IESIs.[15]

To perform a cervical IESI, the patient is placed in a prone position or, if necessary, in a seated or lateral decubitus position. The skin is cleansed with antibacterial solution and the area is draped in a sterile fashion. An AP view of the target region should be obtained (usually C7-T1), with the diameter of the aperture of the interlaminar space optimized, which typically requires tilt of the fluoroscope image intensifier in the caudal direction.

Some physicians prefer a midline approach and others a more lateral or paramedian approach due to the belief that ventral spread of the injectate occurs more reliably with this approach based on investigation performed in the lumbar spine.[40] Yet, studies in both the lumbar and cervical spine show no significant difference in treatment effectiveness between midline and paramedian techniques.[40,41] On proper visualization of the interlaminar space, the target entry point can be planned. The patient is cautioned not to move prior to needle insertion. The skin and superficial subcutaneous tissue are anesthetized directly overlaying the superior edge of the inferior lamina of the target level, slightly off-midline to avoid the spinous process. If the paramedian technique is used, the initial needle target is further lateral on the superior aspect of the inferior lamina of the target level and the final needle tip position lies cephalad to this.

Typically, a 17-gauge to 22-gauge blunt-tip needle (commonly a Tuohy needle) is then introduced. Using guidance with serial fluoroscopic images, using either a contralateral oblique or lateral view to determine needle depth, the needle is advanced toward this initial target until the lamina in touched; this boundary prevents the needle from being inserted too deeply. The needle is then redirected cephalad and toward the midline (for the midline approach) or directly cephalad (for the paramedian approach). At this point a contralateral oblique or lateral fluoroscopic view is reobtained to confirm proper needle depth. The needle is then advanced in submillimeter segments while using loss-of resistance technique to sense the ligamentum flavum density with subsequent loss-of-resistance when the epidural space is encountered. Serial contralateral oblique or lateral views are monitored to confirm depth of needle advance, because loss-of-resistance technique cannot prevent dural puncture with absolute certainty.[39] If appropriate needle-depth is ever in question, advance should be ceased and contrast injected to confirm. Otherwise, once loss of resistance occurs, proper needle tip placement is again assessed on an AP view and either a contralateral oblique or lateral view. If the bevel of the needle should project slightly beyond the anterior margin of the lamina, aspiration is then attempted. Contrast media is then injected and viewed by fluoroscopy, which should demonstrate a characteristic pattern of dispersal confirming epidural placement (**Fig. 3**). At this point, the epidural injectate can be safely deposited.

Contralateral oblique versus lateral view

If the needle is placed at or near midline, lateral radiographic views can gauge depth of insertion based on relation to the silhouette of the lamina. If the needle is placed lateral to midline, the lateral view may exaggerate the actual depth of needle penetration. This can be avoided with a contralateral oblique view in which the beam of the fluoroscope is oriented in parallel to the laminar line where the needle tip lies. This view should depict the lamina against which the tip of the needle lies in cross-section. This contralateral oblique view provides the most accurate depiction of needle depth and should be the view used when making such a determination, particularly if a paramedian approach is used during cervical IESI.[15,42,43]

Additional use of a soft-tipped epidural catheter

In addition to the standard epidural procedure, as outlined previously, the interlaminar approach can also be used to introduce a soft-tipped flexible plastic catheter to more cephalad levels of the cervical epidural space. This method was first described to provide an alternative to the transforaminal approach in delivering steroids to the true site of interest around the pathologic nerve.[15,44] With this technique, the catheter

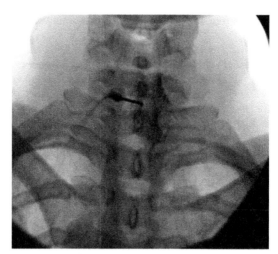

Fig. 3. Right paramedian C7-T1 ESI. The needle tip resides slightly right of midline, as does the Tuohy needle trajectory. Contrast spread is subsequently greater within the epidural space on the right. Characteristic epidural adipose-globules are apparent, and contrast highlights the right lateral recess.

is introduced through a needle inserted at the C7-T1 level or below. The catheter is advanced superiorly until reaching the appropriate level of pathology and can be directed laterally toward the side of pathology in cases of unilateral symptoms (ie, unilateral radicular pain). The ability to directly deposit steroid at a more cranial/lateral site than is accessible via safe interlaminar access at C7-T1 is appealing; randomized controlled study indicates superior pain and functional outcomes associated with use of an epidural catheter versus the standard C7-T1 IESI; however, the study was underpowered to detect a significant difference.[45]

Safety Considerations

The paramount safety concern when performing an interlaminar injection is direct needle injury to the spinal cord. In a review of malpractice claims between 2005 and 2008, there were 64 cases involving cervical interventions, 20 of which resulted in direct spinal cord injury.[46] As previously described, the epidural space is increasingly narrow at higher cervical levels. Given the size of the space, the risk of inadvertently inserting the needle too deep becomes higher at higher cervical levels and can pose a direct risk to the spinal cord. Because of these factors, the Multi-Society Pain Workgroup has recommended that cervical IESIs be performed at the C7-T1 level and preferably no higher than the C6-C7 level.[11] Furthermore, it has been recommended that all cervical interlaminar injections should be performed using image guidance, with appropriate AP, lateral, or contralateral oblique views along with a test dose of contrast medium.[11]

Additionally, anticoagulation status must be determined. In patients who are maintained on therapeutic anticoagulation, continuation versus cessation of anticoagulant and antiplatelet agents has been debated when performing spinal injections that do not use interlaminar access[47,48] due to greater relative consequences of a catastrophic vascular event (ie stroke or myocardial infarction) compared with the possibility of a nonepidural hematoma or other relatively benign bleeding. When using interlaminar access, however, such agents must absolutely be discontinued for sufficient time to restore normal clotting factor and/or platelet function.[49] This is of particular importance when interlaminar access is considered in the cervical spine, where this small space provides minimal reserve for an expanding epidural hematoma before compressive compromise of the spinal cord occurs. If anticoagulation cannot be ceased before cervical IESI, the procedure should not be performed.

Evidence Base for Cervical Epidural Steroid Injections

In the past 5 years, several systematic reviews highlight the strengths and weaknesses apparent in the evidence base for ESI.[5,22,23,29,50–52] One review focuses solely on ESIs performed at cervical levels.[50] This high-quality systematic review noted that all identified randomized controlled trials (RCTs) of cervical TFESIs were unfit for inclusion based on inadequate quality (ie, low ratings for Cochrane review criteria and American Society of Interventional Pain Physician guidelines for RCT reporting). Another comprehensive systematic review focused solely on the evidence base for cervical TFESIs without regard to interlaminar injections.[29] As a whole, cervical IESI studies outnumber investigations of cervical TFESI. Eight RCTs evaluating cervical IESI for numerous indications were identified, although 4 were performed by the same investigator (**Table 1**).[53–56] That said, these studies are notable for their consistency with regard to methodology and outcome measures. In contrast, the evidence base for cervical TFESI comprises observational studies, few of which are prospective in nature (**Table 2**).[57–60]

Methodological heterogeneity limits interpretation of the clinical outcome literature for cervical ESIs. Studies used various definitions of clinical effectiveness in pain reduction, analgesic use, and disability. Pain metrics included numeric rating scale (NRS), the percentage decrease in NRS, proportion of patients with more than 50% improvement in NRS, and similar changes in the visual analog scale (VAS). The reporting of analgesic use was inconsistent among studies (oral morphine equivalents, Medication Quantification Scale Version III). Functional outcome assessment included a variety of measurement tools, including pain disability index (PDI), neck disability index (NDI), Oswestry NDI score, and work status, although with inconsistency among studies.

Cervical IESI has demonstrated durable pain relief and disability improvement for numerous cervical pathologic indications at 12 months to 24 months (see **Table 1**). Numerous factors, however, limit the strength of recommendations for cervical ESIs. As highlighted by Bicket and colleagues,[51] the Achilles heel of the evidence base for cervical ESIs is the lack of placebo control treatment groups. Although Stav and colleagues[61] demonstrated that cervical IESI was superior to posterior cervical intramuscular injections for disk herniation and radiculitis (68% vs 12%). Many any other RCTs followed that used epidural injection of LA, most commonly lidocaine, as the control. The natural concern arises that injection of intramuscular steroid or epidural LA provides more treatment effect than a true placebo.

Whether or not patient selection based on demographic, clinical, or radiologic data influences clinical response to Cervical ESI has not been well studied. Few high-quality studies have sought to identify connections between preinjection data and clinical response. Predictive modeling in 1 RCT demonstrated 2 factors associated with clinical improvement after epidural catheter–directed ILESI: lack of antecedent neck trauma and lower baseline total McGill Pain Questionnaire scores.[45]

Interstudy variability in LA, steroid volume, and steroid concentration used may account for differences in response rate. Furthermore, the duration of benefit for Cervical ESIs is obfuscated by the natural history of cervical pain and radiculopathy. Studies reporting long-term (ie, 1 year) clinical benefit disclosed that injections were repeated several times over the follow-up period (see **Table 1**).[8,45,53,54] No multicenter efforts

Table 1
Studies of the efficacy of cervical interlaminar epidural steroid injections

Study and Design	Indication	Groups and Treatments	Pain Outcomes	Disability Outcomes	Results and Comments
McCormick et al,[45] 2017 RCT, SB	Unilateral radicular pain	1: 40 catheter-targeted IL LA + steroid 2: 40 IL LA + steroid	NRS: improved at 1 and 6 mo for 1 and 2 groups[a] ≥50% % ↓ in NRS: 72% (57–87)[a] vs 60% (45–75)[a] at 1 mo ≥6.8 ↓ in MQS3: 1 mo: 32% vs 25%; 6 mo: 32%[a] vs 39%[a]	OND: improved at 1 and 6 mo[a] PDI: improved at 1 and 6 mo[a]	Epidural catheter-directed IL shows similar efficacy as standard C7-T1 approach IL. Standard approach less fluoroscopy time than catheter-targeted (P<.05) Multiple (2 or 3) injections: 49%
Manchikanti et al,[56] 2014 RCT, DB	Disk herniation and radiculitis	C: 60 IL LA T: 60 IL LA + steroid	NRS: improved at 3, 6, and 12 mo, both groups[b] OME: improved at 3, 6, and 12 mo, C group only[b]	NDI: improved at 3, 6, and 12 mo[b] No difference in work status	Similar efficacy between LA vs LA + steroids Difference in baseline weight between groups, unknown impact Multiple injections: mean 3.5
Manchikanti et al,[66] 2013 RCT, DB	Disk herniation	C: 60 IL LA T: 60 IL LA + steroid	NRS: improved at 3, 6, 12, and 24 mo, both groups¥ OME: improved at 3, 6, 12, and 24 mo, both groups¥	NDI: improved at 3, 6, 12, and 24 mo, both groups¥ No difference in work status	Similar efficacy between LA vs LA + steroids Difference in baseline weight between groups, unknown impact Multiple injections: mean 5–6
Manchikanti et al,[65] 2012 RCT, DB	Cervical spinal stenosis	C: 30 IL LA T: 30 IL LA + steroid	NRS: improved at 3, 6, and 12 mo, both groups¥ OME: improved at 3, 6, and 12 mo, both groups¥	NDI:improved at 3, 6, and 12 mo, both groups¥ No difference in work status	Similar efficacy between LA vs LA + steroids. Difference in baseline weight between groups, unknown impact Multiple injections: mean 3–4

Study	Condition	Groups	Pain outcomes	Functional outcomes	Comments
Manchikanti et al,[53] 2012 RCT, DB	Cervical postsurgery syndrome	C: 28 IL LA T: 28 IL LA + steroid	NRS: improved at 3, 6, and 12 mo OME: no improvement at 3, 6, and 12 mo, either group	NDI: mproved at 3, 6, and 12 mo, both groups¥ No difference in work status	Similar efficacy between LA vs LA + steroids Difference in gender proportion and height between groups, unknown impact Multiple injections: mean 3.5
Pasqualucci et al,[63] 2007 RCT, UB	Unilateral cervicobrachial pain without prior cervical spine surgery	1: single-shot IL LA + steroid 2: continuous IL LA + steroid	% ↓ in VAS 1 mo:59% ± 21% vs 75% ± 15%; 6 mo: 58% ± 23% vs 74% ± 16% Hours pain-free sleep: improved at 1 and 6 mo, both groups[a]	NR	Only in patients with pain duration >9 mo are continuous epidural superior to single-shot IL No fluoroscopy used
Castagnera et al,[64] 1994 RCT, SB	Disk herniation and radiculitis	C: 14 IL LA + steroid T: 10 LA + steroid + morphine	≥50% ↓ in VAS (groups merged): 3 mo: 67%; 6 mo: 71%; 12 mo: 71%	No difference in work status	Epidural morphine (2.5 mg) does not improve outcomes when combined with LA + steroid. Side effects from epidural morphine noted, but not quantified. No fluoroscopy used
Stav et al,[61] 1993 RCT, UB	Disk herniation and radiculitis	C: 17 posterior neck muscle LA + steroid T: 25 IL LA + steroid	% ↓ in VAS 12 mo: 12% vs 56% (P<.05) ↓ in analgesic use 12 mo: 9% vs 64% (P<.05)	ROM: 1 y: ~10% vs ~70% (P<.05) Work status at 1 y: 6% vs 61% (P<.05)	Cervical ESIs are superior to posterior neck muscle injection. Multiple injections: mean 2.5 No fluoroscopy used

Outcomes are reported as, percentage (95% confidence interval), mean ± SEM, or median [interquartile range] unless otherwise stated.

Abbreviations: C, control group; DB, double-blinded; IL, interlaminar; mo, month; MQS3, Medication Quantification Scale Version III; NR, not reported; OME, oral morphine equivalents; ONDI, Oswestry NDI score; ROM, range of motion; SB, single-blinded; T, treatment; UB, unblinded.

[a] P<.05 versus baseline.

[b] P<.01 versus baseline, ¥P<.001 versus baseline.

Table 2
Studies of the efficacy of cervical transforaminal epidural steroid injections

Study and Design	Indication	Groups and Treatments	Pain Outcomes	Disability Outcomes	Results and Comments
Lee and Lee,[59] 2016 PCS, UB	Disk herniation or spinal stenosis. Partial responders (NRS >4) after prior TF.	C: 76 TF (LA + steroid) T: 108 (LA + steroid)	Duration NRS <3 (in mo): 6.2 ± 2.9 vs 9.7 ± 2.2¥	NR	Raw NRS values not reported Scheduled repeat injections 2 w may decrease overall utilization in 1 y.
Lee and Lee,[58] 2011 RCT, UB	Disk herniation with >3 mo radiculopathy without stenosis	C: 65 TF (LA + steroid) under C-arm T: 51 TF (LA + steroid) under CT	≥50% ↓ in NRS at 2 mo: Arm pain: 55% vs 73%[a] Neck pain: 58% vs 73%	Korean NDI at 2 mo: 58% vs 76%[a]	CT guidance may be superior to C-arm guidance Substantial increase in radiation exposure for CT vs fluoroscopy
Persson and Anderberg,[60] 2012 PCS, UB	Radiculitis from stenosis with prior 50% response to diagnostic SNRB	140 TF	≥50% ↓ in VAS at 14 w: 49%	NDI: significant ↓ only in cohort with ≥50% ↓ in VAS	Short follow-up period LA and steroid dose and agent not reported Multiple injections: 3-w interval
Andenberg et al,[57] 2007 RCT	Unilateral radiculitis	C: 20 LA + saline T: 20 LA + steroid	≥50% ↓ in VAS at 2 w: 30%	NR	Underpowered study, short follow-up period

Outcomes are reported as, percentage (95% CI), mean ± SEM, or median (interquartile range), unless otherwise stated.
Abbreviations: C, control group; DB, double-blinded; mo, month; NR, not reported; PCS, prospective cohort study; SB, single-blinded; SNRB, single nerve root block; T, treatment group; UB, unblended.
[a] $P<.05$, ¥$P<.001$.

are reported in the literature. The Spine Intervention Society and the American Academy of Physical Medicine and Rehabilitation recommendation 2 weeks between repeat ESIs for concerns of assessing efficacy and minimizing the risk of adrenal suppression with multiple corticosteroid deliveries.[15,62]

SUMMARY

Cervical ESIs are among the most common interventional pain procedures performed for radicular pain. Important safety considerations include attention to the possibility of spinal cord infarction and spinal epidural hematoma. When appropriate radiographic, technical, and pharmacologic principals are used, these procedures are relatively safe. Cervical ESIs provide fairly effective short-term treatment effect. Long-term outcomes, however, are less certain. The evidence base for cervical ESIs is limited by methodological heterogeneity and lack of comparison to a true placebo group.

REFERENCES

1. Cohen S. Epidemiology, diagnosis, and treatment of neck pain. Mayo Clin Proc 2015;90(2):284–99.
2. Fejer R, Kyvik K, Hartvigsen J. The prevalence of neck pain in the world population: a systematic critical review of the literature. Eur Spine J 2006;15(6):834–48.
3. Iyer S, Kim H. Cervical radiculopathy. Curr Rev Musculoskelet Med 2016;9: 272–80.
4. Van Boxem K, Huntoon M, Van Zundert J, et al. Pulsed radiogrequency: a review of the basic science as applied to the pathophysiology of radicular pain: a call for clinical translation. Reg Anesth Pain Med 2014;39(2):149–59.
5. Mattie R, McCormick Z, Yu S, et al. Are all epidurals created equally? a systematic review of the literature on caudal, interlaminar, and transforaminal injections from the last 5 years. Curr Phys Med Rehabil Rep 2015;3(2):159–72.
6. Radhakrishnan K, Litchy W, O'Fallon W, et al. Epidemiology of cervical radiculopathy. A population-based student from Rochester, Minnesota, 1976 through 1990. Brain 1994;117(2):325–35.
7. Woods B, Hilibrand A. Cervical radiculopathy: epidemiology, etiology, diagnosis, and treatment. J Spinal Disord Tech 2015;28:251.
8. Manchikanti L, Pampati V, Hirsch J. Retrospective cohort study of usage patterns of epidural injections for spinal pain in the US fee-for-service Medicare population from 2000 to 2014. BMJ Open 2016;6(12):e013042.
9. Friedly J, Chan L, Deyo R. Geographic variation in epidural steroid injection use in medicare patients. J Bone Joint Surg Am 2008;90(8):1730–7.
10. Bosmia A, Hogan E, Loukas M, et al. Blood supply to the human spinal cord: part I. Anatomy and hemodynamics. Clin Anat 2015;28(1):52–64.
11. Rathmell J, Benzon H, Dreyfuss P, et al. Safeguards to prevent neurologic complications after epidural steroid injectionsconsensus opinions from a multidisciplinary working group and national organizations. Anesthesiology 2015;122(5): 974–84.
12. Hoeft M, Rathmell J, Monsey R, et al. Cervical transforaminal injection and the radicular artery: variation in anatomical location within the cervical intervertebral foramina. Reg Anesth Pain Med 2006;31(3):270–4.
13. Huntoon M. Anatomy of the cervical intervertebral foramina: vulnerable arteries and ischemic neurologic injuries after transforaminal epidural injections. Pain 2005;117(1–2):104–11.

14. Sullivan W, Willick S, Chira-Adisai W, et al. Incidence of intravas- cular uptake in lumbar spinal injection procedures. Spine 2000;25(4):481–6.

15. Bogduk N. Practice guidelines for spinal diagnostic and treatment procedures. 2nd edition. San Francisco: International Spine Intervention Society; 2013.

16. Schneider B, Zheng P, Mattie R, et al. Safety of epidural steroid injections. Expert Opin Drug Saf 2016;15(8):1031–9.

17. Carr C, Plastaras C, Pingree M, et al. Immediate adverse events in interventional pain procedures: a multi-institutional study. Pain Med 2016;17(12):2155–61.

18. Bose B. Quadriparesis following cervical epidural steroid injections: case report and review of the literature. Spine J 2005;5(5):558–63.

19. Kennedy D, Dreyfuss P, Aprill C, et al. Paraplegia following image-guided trans- foraminal lumbar spine epidural steroid injection: two case reports. Pain Med 2009;10(8):1389–94.

20. Okubadejo G, Talcott M, Schmidt R, et al. Perils of intravascular methylprednisolone injection into the vertebral artery: an animal study. J Bone Joint Surg Am 2005;90(9):1932–8.

21. Derby R, Lee SH, Date E, et al. Size and aggregation of corticosteroids used for epidural injections. Pain Med 2008;9(2):227–34.

22. Mehta P, Syrop I, Singh J, et al. Systematic review of the efficacy of particulate versus nonparticulate corticosteroids in epidural injections. PM R 2017;9(5): 502–12.

23. Feeley I, Healy E, Noel J, et al. Particulate and non-particulate steroids in spinal epidurals: a systematic review and meta-analysis. Eur Spine J 2017;26(2): 336–44.

24. McCormick Z, Cushman D, Marshall B, et al. Pain reduction and repeat injections after transforaminal epidural injection with particulate versus nonparticulate steroid for the treatment of chronic painful lumbosacral radiculopathy. PM R 2016; 8(11):1039–45.

25. El-Yahchouchi C, Geske J, Carter R, et al. The noninferiority of the nonparticulate steroid dexamethasone vs the particulate steroids betamethasone and triamcinolone in lumbar transforaminal epidural steroid injections. Pain Med 2013;14(11): 1650–7.

26. Kennedy D, Plastaras C, Casey E, et al. Comparative effectiveness of lumbar transforaminal epidural steroid injections with particulate versus nonparticulate corticosteroids for lumbar radicular pain due to intervertebral disc herniation: a prospective, randomized, double-blind trial. Pain Med 2014;15(4):548–55.

27. Denis I, Claveau G, Filiatrault M, et al. Randomized double-blind controlled trial comparing the effectiveness of lumbar transforaminal epidural injections of particulate and nonparticulate corticosteroids for lumbosacral radicular pain. Pain Med 2015;16(9):1697–708.

28. Collighan N, Gupta S, Richardson J, et al. Re: Comparison of the effectiveness of lumbar transforaminal epidural injection with the particulate and nonparticulate corticosteroids in lumbar radiating pain. Pain Med 2011;12(8):1290–1.

29. Engel A, King W, MacVicar J. Society; SDotISI. The effectiveness and risks of fluoroscopically guided cervical transforaminal injections of steroids: a systematic review with comprehensive analysis of the published data. Pain Med 2014;15(3): 386–402.

30. Chung S. Convulsion caused by a lidocaine test in cervical transforaminal epidural steroid injection. PM R 2011;3(7):674–7.

31. Schellhas K, Pollei S, Johnson B, et al. Selective cervical nerve root blockade: experience with a safe and reliable technique using an anterolateral approach for needle placement. AJNR Am J Neuroradiol 2007;28(10):1909–14.

32. Hwang H, Park J, Lee W, et al. Crystallization of local anesthetics when mixed with corticosteroid solutions. Ann Rehabil Med 2016;40(1):21–7.

33. Jasper J. Role of digital subtraction fluoroscopic imaging in detecting intravascular injections. Pain Physician 2003;6(3):369–72.

34. McLean J, Sigler J, Plastaras C, et al. The rate of detection of intravascular injection in cervical transforaminal epidural steroid injections with and without digital subtraction angiography. PM R 2009;1(7):636–42.

35. Chang Chien G, Candido K, Knezevic N. Digital subtraction angiography does not reliably prevent paraplegia associated with lumbar transforaminal epidural steroid injection. Pain Physician 2012;15(6):515–23.

36. Maus T, Schueler B, Leng S, et al. Radiation dose incurred in the exclusion of vascular filling in transforaminal epidural steroid injections: fluoroscopy, digital subtraction angiography, and CT/fluoroscopy. Pain Med 2014;15(8):1328–33.

37. Mukerji N, Todd N. Spinal epidural haematoma; factors influencing outcome. Br J Neurosurg 2013;27(6):712–7.

38. Hogan Q. Epidural anatomy examined by cryomicrotome section. Influence of age, vertebral level, and disease. Reg Anesth 1996;21(5):395–406.

39. Stojanovic M, Vu T, Caneris O, et al. The role of fluoroscopy in cervical epidural steroid injections: an analysis of contrast dispersal patterns. Spine (Phila Pa 1976) 2002;1(27):509–14.

40. Gupta R, Singh S, Kaur S, et al. Correlation between epidurographic contrast flow patterns and clinical effectiveness in chronic lumbar discogenic radicular pain treated with epidural steroid injections via different approaches. Korean J Pain 2014;27(4):353–9.

41. Yoon J, Kwon J, Yoon Y, et al. Cervical interlaminar epidural steroid injection for unilateral cervical radiculopathy: comparison of midline and paramedian approaches for efficacy. Korean J Radiol 2015;16(3):604–12.

42. Gill J, Aner M, Nagda J, et al. Contralateral oblique view is superior to lateral view for interlaminar cervical and cervicothoracic epidural access. Pain Med 2015;16(1):68–80.

43. Landers M, Dreyfuss P, Bogduk N. On the geometry of fluoroscopy views for cervical interlaminar epidural injections. Pain Med 2012;13(1):58–65.

44. Larkin T, Carragee E, Cohen S. A novel technique for delivery of epidural steroids and diagnosing the level of nerve root pathology. J Spinal Disord Tech 2003;16(2):186–92.

45. McCormick Z, Nelson A, Bhave M, et al. A prospective randomized comparative trial of targeted steroid injection via epidural catheter versus standard C7-T1 interlaminar approach for the treatment of unilateral cervical radicular pain. Reg Anesth Pain Med 2017;42(1):82–9.

46. Rathmell J, Michna E, Fitzgibbon D, et al. Injury and liability associated with cervical procedures for chronic pain. Anesthesiol 2011;114(4):918–26.

47. Goodman B, House L, Vallabhaneni S, et al. Anticoagulant and antiplatelet management for spinal procedures: a prospective, descriptive study. Pain Med 2017;18(7):1218–24.

48. Endres S, Shufelt A, Bogduk N. The risks of continuing or discontinuing anticoagulants for patients undergoing common interventional pain procedures. Pain Med 2017;18(3):403–9.

49. Narouze S, Benzon H, Provenzano D, et al. Interventional spine and pain procedures in patients on antiplatelet and anticoagulant medications: guidelines from the American Society of Regional Anesthesia and Pain Medicine, the European Society Of Regional Anaesthesia And Pain Therapy, the American academy of pain medicine, the International Neuromodulation Society, the North American Neuromodulation Society, and the World Institute of Pain. Reg Anesth Pain Med 2015;40(3):182–212.
50. Manchikant L, Nampiaparampil D, Candido K, et al. Do cervical epidural injections provide long-term relief in neck and upper extremity pain? a systematic review. Pain Physician 2015;18(1):39–60.
51. Bicket M, Gupta A, Brown CT, et al. Epidural injections for spinal pain: a systematic review and meta-analysis evaluating the "control" injections in randomized controlled trials. Anesthesiol 2016;119(4):907–31.
52. Cohen S, Bicket M, Jamison D, et al. Epidural steroids: a comprehensive, evidence-based review. Reg Anesth Pain Med 2013;38(3):175–200.
53. Manchikanti L, Malla Y, Cash K, et al. Fluoroscopic cervical interlaminar epidural injections in managing chronic pain of cervical postsurgery syndrome: preliminary results of a randomized, double-blind, active control trial. Pain Physician 2012;15:13–5.
54. Manchikanti L, Cash K, Pampati V, et al. Cervical epidural injections in chronic discogenic neck pain without disc herniation or radiculitis: preliminary results of a randomized, double-blind, controlled trial. Pain Physician 2010;13:E265–78.
55. Manchikanti L, Cash K, Pampati V, et al. The effectiveness of fluoroscopic cervical interlaminar epidural injections in managing chronic cervical disc herniation and radiculitis: prliminary results of a randomize, double-blind, controlled trial. Pain Physician 2010;13:223–36.
56. Manchikanti L, Cash K, Pampati V, et al. Two-year follow-up results of fluoroscopic cervical epidural injections in chronic axial or discogenic neck pain: a randomized, double-blind, controlled trial. Int J Med Sci 2014;11(4):309–20.
57. Anderberg L, Annertz M, Persson L, et al. Transforaminal steroid injections for the treatment of cervical radiculopathy: a prospective and randomised study. Eur Spine J 2007;16(3):321–8.
58. Lee J, Lee S. Comparison of clinical effectiveness of cervical transforaminal steroid injection according to different radiological guidances (C-arm fluoroscopy vs. computed tomography fluoroscopy). Spine J 2011;11(5):416–23.
59. Lee J, Lee S. Can repeat injection provide clinical benefit in patients with cervical disc herniation and stenosis when the first epidural injection results only in partial response? Medicine (Baltimore) 2016;95(29):e4131.
60. Persson L, Anderberg L. Repetitive transforaminal steroid injections in cervical radiculopathy: a prospective outcome study including 140 patients. Evid Based Spine Care J 2012;3(3):13–20.
61. Stav A, Ovadia L, Sternberg A, et al. Cervical epidural steroid injection for cervicobrachialgia. Acta Anaesthesiol Scand 1993;37:562–6.
62. Casazza B, Chou L, Davis S, et al. Educational guidelines for interventional spinal procedures. 2008.
63. Pasqualucci A, Varrassi G, Braschi A, et al. Epidural local anesthetic plus corticosteroid for the treatment of cervical brachial radicular pain: single injection versus continuous infusion. Clin J Pain 2007;23(7):551–7.
64. Castagnera L, Maurette P, Pointillart V, et al. Long-term results of cervical epidural steroid injection with and without morphine in chronic cervical radicular pain. Pain 1994;58(2):239–43.

65. Manchikanti L, Malla Y, Cash KA, et al. Fluoroscopic epidural injections in cervical spinal stenosis: preliminary results of a randomized, double-blind, active control trial. Pain Physician 2012;15(1):E59–70.
66. Manchikanti L, Cash KA, Pampati V, et al. A randomized, double-blind, active control trial of fluoroscopic cervical interlaminar epidural injections in chronic pain of cervical disc herniation: results of a 2-year follow-up. Pain Physician 2013;16(5):465–78.

Image and Contrast Flow Pattern Interpretation for Attempted Epidural Steroid Injections

Michael B. Furman, MD, MS[a,b,c],*, Anthony A. Cuneo, MD, PhD[d]

KEYWORDS

- Contrast flow patterns • Interventional spine procedures • Epidural steroid injections
- Epidural contrast flow • Subarachnoid contrast flow

KEY POINTS

- Identifying and recognizing the significance of different contrast flow patterns is an integral component of performing interventional spinal procedures.
- The practitioner should be aware of the distinct patterns discussed and be able to identify them and react accordingly.
- Recognizing the potential complications in the various spaces discussed and appreciating the gravity of suboptimally placed epidural injections are instrumental in providing safe and effective procedures.

Fluoroscopically guided, contrast-enhanced epidural steroid injections (ESIs) are frequently performed for radicular symptoms. Interventionalists performing these procedures should have a thorough and detailed understanding of spinal anatomy to safely and effectively deliver the desired injectate to the targeted site. Contrast dye flow patterns visualized with real-time fluoroscopy provide invaluable guidance for decision making prior to placing the final injectate.[1,2] Being able to differentiate epidural from nonepidural contrast flow is vitally important. In addition, recognizing flow to undesired locations is equally, if not more imperative. This article summarizes the characteristics that distinguish between ideal epidural flow patterns and nonideal subarachnoid, intradural, and other suboptimal contrast flow patterns. Recognizing these patterns is essential for safe and successful ESIs and to prevent avoidable complications.

The author has nothing to disclose.
[a] Interventional Spine and Sports, OSS Health, York, PA, USA; [b] Rehabilitation Medicine, Sinai Hospital, Baltimore, MD, USA; [c] Physical Medicine and Rehabilitation, Temple University School of Medicine, Philadelphia, PA, USA; [d] Interventional Pain Management Physician, The Orthopedic Group, 1145 Bower Hill Road #301, Pittsburgh, PA 15243, USA
* Physical Medicine and Rehabilitation, Temple University School of Medicine, 3500 N Broad Street, Philadelphia, PA 19140.
E-mail address: mbfurman@gmail.com

Adverse outcomes and unfavorable consequences can occur from inadvertent non-epidural injections. The most serious adverse outcomes include paralysis, stroke, and death. Correctly interpreting and distinguishing between expected and suboptimal contrast flow patterns will prevent almost all potential negative sequelae.

Most interventionalists can recognize ideal epidural contrast flow. However, analyzing contrast patterns in the context of pathologically deranged anatomy and distinguishing undesirable spread require the ability to perform a 3-dimensional spatial reconstruction from a 2-dimensional fluoroscopic image. Of paramount importance is the ability to incorporate this anatomic knowledge as a needle is advanced toward the desired target, and knowing when delivery of injectate could result in adverse outcomes.

There are unique flow patterns that can be encountered with attempted interlaminar versus transforaminal approaches. With a transforaminal injection, the injectate could enter the extraforaminal or fascial space, the desired epidural space, intraneural space, intradural space, or subarachnoid space (ordered from most dorsolateral to ventromedial). With an interlaminar injection, the needle can pass midline or paramedian through the soft tissue/fascia, ligamentum flavum, epidural space, intradural space, and/or subarachnoid spaces (ordered from most dorsal to ventral). Other areas of potential suboptimal injection include intravascular, retrodural space of Okada, intra-articular facet, and intradiscal, all of which will also be discussed. Of note, epidural injections via a caudal approach are not addressed in this article.

EPIDURAL CONTRAST FLOW

For ease of comparison and discussion, the normal, optimal epidural contrast flow will be discussed and described first (**Figs. 1** and **2**, **Table 1**). The epidural space is a potential space. The desired epidural contrast flow in an anterior- posterior (AP) projection has vacuolization and tends to be asymmetric, even lateralizing to one side at times. The contrast will contact the medial pedicle on the side of the procedure, especially for injections with a transforaminal approach. Live injection should ideally be nonvascular. Contralateral oblique (CLO) imaging to the needle tip should have a uniform spread immediately ventral to the ventral interlaminar line (VILL) which is visualized along the lamina's ventral margins.[3] On lateral projection, the contrast will be in a uniform line, appreciated immediately ventral to the spinolaminar line which is visualized along the bases of the spinous processes. Only after recognizing and confirming

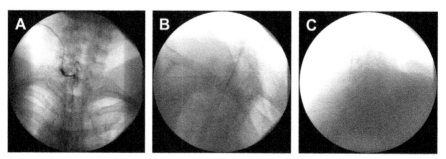

Fig. 1. Demonstrates the epidural contrast pattern seen in a cervical interlaminar epidural steroid injection. (*A*) AP view: note asymmetric vacuolization appearance of the contrast flow. (*B*) CLO view: note the contrast flow directly ventral to the ventral interlaminar line. (*C*) Lateral view: note the contrast flow directly ventral to the spinolaminar line.

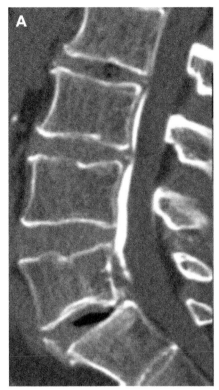
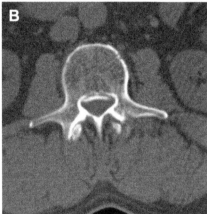

Fig. 2. Sagital and axial CT after lumbar transformainal epidural steroid injection. (*A*) Sagittal midline CT. (*B*) Axial CT. Note the nonuniform flow localized directly ventral to the vertebral body. (*Courtesy of* Tim Maus, MD, Mayo Clinic, Rochester, MN.)

the correct contrast flow pattern should one proceed with the final injectate administration targeted for the epidural space.

SUBARACHNOID CONTRAST FLOW

The subarachnoid (intrathecal) space is the target location when performing a myelogram (**Figs. 3** and **4**; see **Table 1**). However, a subarachnoid injection is an undesired complication of epidural steroid injections. In AP projection, contrast injection into the intrathecal space will demonstrate an hourglass symmetric flow pattern. The contrast crosses midline and spreads left to right and rostral to caudal diffusely. An AP alone may be too insensitive to detect intrathecal flow, leading to a possible false-negative intrathecal contrast pattern, often confused with an epidural injection. This unrecognized scenario is a source of potential harm to the patient if the final injectate is placed intrathecally.

Even with small contrast volumes, oblique and lateral views will demonstrate layering in a gravitationally dependent portion of the thecal sac. This generates a fluid-fluid (cerebrospinal fluid [CSF]-contrast dye) level, forming a straight posterior margin. Puncturing of the intrathecal space can cause spinal headaches, while injection of anesthetic and steroid can lead to mild transient symptoms such as paresthesias and arachnoiditis, or more morbid conditions such as meningitis, cauda

Table 1
Contrast flow pattern characteristics appreciated in different fluoroscopic projections

	AP Characteristics	CLO Characteristics	Lateral Characteristics	Potential Injection Outcome
Epidural (optimal)	• Vacuolization • Often asymmetric • Contrast contacts medial pedicle (especially with TFESI)	• Contrast contacts immediately ventral to the lamina along the VILL when the needle tip is contralateral	• Uniform line immediately ventral to the spinolaminar line • Ventral contrast uniformly contacts VB	• Improvement
Subarachnoid (intrathecal)	• Crosses midline • Symmetric • Contrast does not contact medial pedicle	• Distinct fluid-fluid (CSF-contrast dye) level, with the distinct ventral dye layering dependently • Contrast does not contact the VILL	• Hazy dorsal fluid-fluid (CSF-contrast dye) level, with the distinct ventral dye layering dependently • Contrast does not contact the VB	• Spinal headache • Sensory and/or motor block including paresthesias, cauda equina or conus medularis syndrome • Arachnoiditis or meningitis
Intradural (subdural) – cystic-like pattern	• Narrow pillar form • Asymmetric or Unilateral • Distinct boundaries • Uniform dense appearance • Sharp margination • Contrast does not contact medial pedicle	• Contrast does not contact the VILL	• Contrast can spread dorsal or ventral but does not contact VB	• Painful injection
Intradural (subdural) – dural boundary layer pattern	• Symmetric, bilateral • Contrast approximates medial pedicle but does not exit foramina • Tram tracks	• Contrast approximates the VILL	• Extensive narrow, linear column extending cephalad • Contrast dorsal and ventral • Does not consistently contact VB	• Painful injection • Sensory and/or motor block • Autonomic nervous system depression leading to hemodynamic instability and respiratory paralysis
Fascial (extradural)	• Localized and possibly spreading along fascia layers • Contrast does not contact medial pedicle	• Localized contrast dorsal to VILL	• Localized contrast dorsal to spinolaminar line	• No improvement

Abbreviations: CLO, contralateral oblique; ILESI, Interlaminar epidural steroid injection; TFESI, transforaminal epidural steroid injection; VB, vertebral body; VILL, ventral interlaminar line.

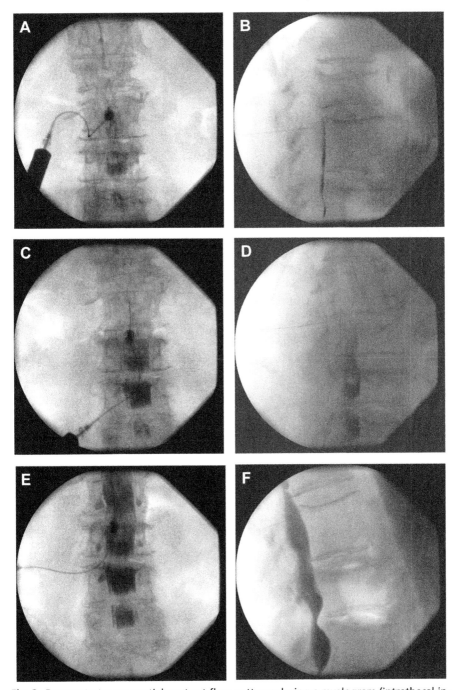

Fig. 3. Demonstrates sequential contrast flow patterns during a myelogram (intrathecal injection) with an L1-2 midline needle placement. There is margination ventrally and a fluid interface dorsally. (*A, B*) Initial AP and lateral views of the myelogram. (*C, D*) AP and CLO views during the midway point of the myelogram. (*E, F*) Final AP and lateral views of the myelogram. Especially note the initial intrathecal injection patterns (see *A* and *B*) when low contrast volumes are injected.

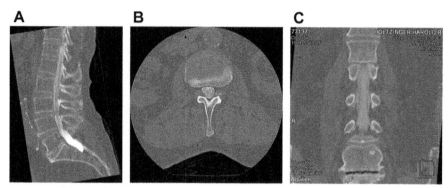

Fig. 4. CT after myelogram injection. (*A*) Midline sagittal view. (*B*) Axial view. (*C*) Coronal view. Note the uniform dye pattern and the small thin space surrounding the contrast, representing the dura and epidural space.

equina, or conus medullaris syndrome. The symptomatology will depend on the level of penetration, degree of blockade, and contents of the injectate.

INTRADURAL CONTRAST FLOW

The intradural (subdural) space is also a potential space. There are 2 subdural/intradural space injection patterns that can be appreciated: cystic-like and dural boundary layer.

Cystic-Like Intradural Injections

For cystic-like intradural injections, contrast flow can appear as localized accumulation of contrast medium at the periphery of the meningeal tube with sharp, often undulating margins (**Figs. 5** and **6**; see **Table 1**). There is typically radial expansion, rather than longitudinal spread of contrast, displacing the arachnoid centrally and acting as a mass that can potentially cause neural compression and often causing pain. CLO and lateral views can demonstrate contrast spreading dorsal and ventral, but it will not contact the VILL in CLO projection or spinolaminal line or VB in lateral projection. Mixed compartment patterns are often present with epidural and subarachnoid contrast accompanying intradural flow, adding to the diagnostic challenge. Oftentimes, the contrast can be reaspirated into the syringe after these injections.

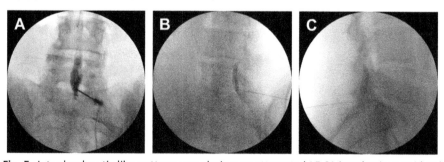

Fig. 5. Intradural cystic-like pattern seen during an attempted L5-S1 interlaminar epidural steroid injection. (*A*) AP view with sharp margination of intradural/subdural flow. Contrast injection caused the patient discomfort. (*B*) CLO view of intradural/subdural flow in the same patient. Note the sharp margination of contrast flow. (*C*) Lateral view of intradural flow in the same patient.

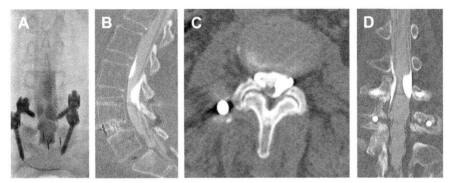

Fig. 6. Mixed intrathecal and cystic-like subdural/intradural injection encountered during myelography. (*A*) AP fluoroscopy. (*B*) Midline sagittal CT. (*C*) CT axial. (*D*) Coronal CT. Note the denser contrast and sharp margination to the subdural cystic component compared with the intrathecal/subarachnoid contrast. (*Courtesy of* Tim Maus, MD, Mayo Clinic, Rochester, MN.)

Dural Boundary Layer Intradural Injections

The classic description of intradural flow associated with ascending anesthetic blocks or respiratory compromise is where contrast is observed concentrically within the wall of the meningeal tube giving a train track appearance as demonstrated in **Fig. 7**A.[4–6] This represents creation of a subdural cleavage plane at the dural border cell level. When cleavage is widespread, contrast distributes in a thin, nonuniform sheet, most easily seen with a CLO or lateral view. The contrast will localize to the ventral or dorsal margins (**Figs. 7 and 8**). The contrast will appear dense and potentially spread along spinal nerve sleeves, potentially mimicking epidural flow. However, intradural flow typically does not exit the formina, while epidural flow does.

  Fig. 9 presents side-by-side comparisons of Fluoroscopic and computed tomography (CT) images of these different contrast patterns for an even better appreciation.

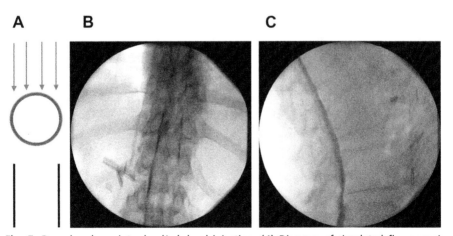

Fig. 7. Boundary layer intradural/subdural injection. (*A*) Diagram of simulated fluoroscopic beam (*arrows*) shooting through boundary layer subdural or intraneural contrast (*circle*). The resultant pattern seen on fluoroscopy is represented by the 2 black lines, which appear as parallel train tracks. (*B*) AP and (*C*) initial lateral fluoroscopic injection of attempted myelography resulting in subdural/intradural flow pattern. Subsequent corresponding CT images are seen in **Fig. 8**.

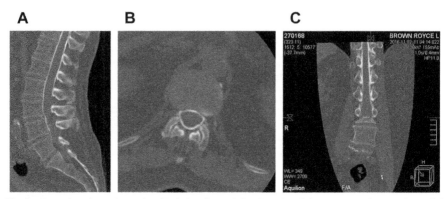

Fig. 8. Boundary layer intradural/subdural postinjection CT of the same patient as in A. (*A*) Midline sagittal CT. (*B*) CT axial CT. (*C*) Coronal CT. Note the bright uniform contrast pattern surrounding the dark intrathecal/subarachnoid space.

FASCIAL CONTRAST FLOW

Identifying fascial (extradural) contrast flow is relatively straightforward. The contrast tends to localize within/along the dorsal fascial planes with limited caudal and rostral migration (**Fig. 10**; see **Table 1**). Contrast will not contact the medial pedicle on AP view. CLO or lateral imaging will localize contrast dorsal to the VILL or spinolaminar line, respectively. When this flow pattern and location are seen, harm to the patient is unlikely; however, a desired successful injection is also unlikely. The interventionalist should reposition the needle to achieve the desired epidural flow pattern.

VASCULAR CONTRAST FLOW

Finding blood in the needle hub after aspiration is 97% specific, but only 46% sensitive when attempting to identify intravascular needle placement.[6–8] Identification of intravascular needle placement can be greatly improved with live contrast injection (**Fig. 11**). Intravascular flow can be recognized in 19.4% of cervical and 11.2% of lumbar transforaminal epidural injections with live contrast injection. Identification of intravascular flow will be even more evident with live contrast injection using digital subtraction.[9–11] The contrast will demonstrate a serpiginous, nonlinear pattern that dissipates quickly. Certain characteristics may potentially help distinguish between venous and arterial flow patterns (**Table 2**). The interventionalist should abort the procedure for arterial flow, while the needle can be repositioned for venous flow. Of note, placement of injectate in the arterial system has the potential to cause spinal cord infarction or stroke depending on the injectate composition and the location of the procedure.

RETRODURAL SPACE OF OKADA CONTRAST FLOW

Interventionalists should also be able to recognize contrast flow into the retrodural space of Okada.[12] This space can provide communication between neighboring facet joints, dorsal to the ligamentum flavum in the interlaminar zone (**Fig. 12**). Contrast can be seen spreading from 1 facet joint across midline to the contralateral facet joint. Injecting in to this space would be nonideal for a targeted epidural injection, and the needle should be repositioned.

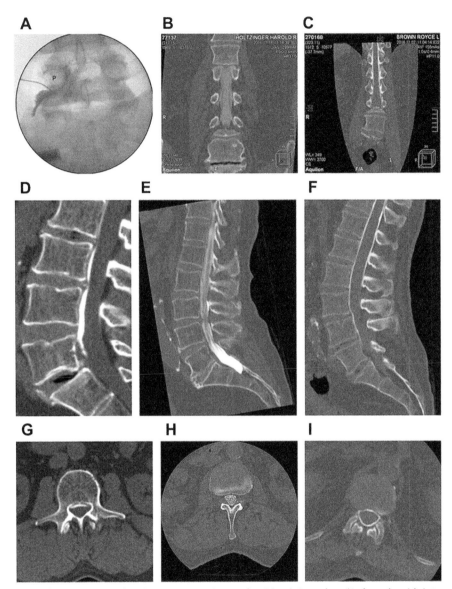

Fig. 9. Fluoroscopic and CT image comparisons of epidural, intrathecal/subarachnoid, intra-dural/subdural space-dural boundary cell layer, respectively. (*A–C*) Coronal images for compar-ison to each other. (*A*) AP fluoroscopic image of left L5 transformainal ESI with contrast exiting below the pedicle (P). (*B*) Coronal CT of myelogram demonstrating subarachnoid/intra-thecal contrast. (*C*) Coronal CT of subdural contrast flow. Note that contrast does not appear distal to the foramina with an intradural/subdural or intrathecal space injection. Epidural space contrast can be seen exiting the foramina in A. (*D–F*) Sagital CT images for comparison to each other. (*D*) Midline sagittal CT of epidural flow (*E*) midline sagittal CT myelogram demonstrating subarachnoid/intrathecal contrast. (*F*) Midline sagittal CT of subdural/intra-dural boundary cell layer contrast flow. The sagittal images demonstrate diffuse spread of contrast with both intrathecal and intradural boundary cell layer space injections, while the epidural space injection remains localized. Note the black space ventral and dorsal to the myelogram in E representing the dura/epidural space. There is a train tracks appearance with the intradural space injection. Epidural space contrast can be seen abutting the VB.

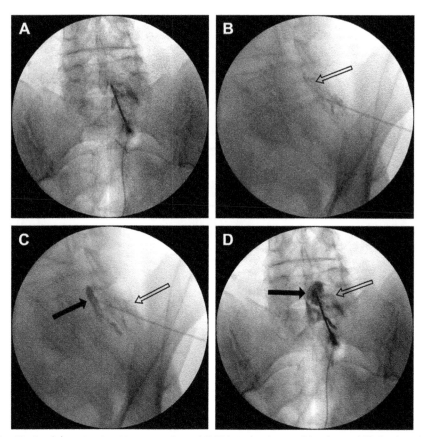

Fig. 10. Fascial contrast pattern seen in an L5-S1 interlaminar epidural steroid injection. (*A*) AP view with questionable epidural flow. (*B*) CLO view confirms that the contrast flow is extradural (*open arrow*). Note that the suboptimal contrast is localized dorsal to the ventral interlaminar line. (*C*) CLO view in the same patient after repositioning the needle with a true loss of resistance demonstrating optimal epidural contrast flow (*closed arrow*). Note the previously seen extradural flow for comparison (*open arrow*). (*D*) AP view in the same patient with both epidural (*closed arrow*) and extradural (*open arrow*) contrast flows.

INTRA-ARTICULAR FACET CONTRAST FLOW

Inadvertent facet joint placement of contrast with an attempted epidural injection can be seen, especially with a transforaminal approach. Often the needle tip is not ventral enough and/or strays too far medially and remains within the capsule of the neighboring facet joint. Contrast flow will have a vertical-inferior pattern localized outside of the

---

(*G–I*) Axial CT images for comparison with each other. (*G*) Axial CT of epidural flow. (*H*) Axial CT myelogram demonstrating subarachnoid/intrathecal contrast. (*I*) Axial CT of subdural contrast flow. The axial images demonstrate diffuse spread of contrast with both intrathecal and intradural boundary cell layer space injections, while the epidural space injection remains localized. Note the black space surrounding the myelogram in H representing the dura/epidural space. Nerves are visualized with injection of the intrathecal space with contrast. The intradural boundary cell layer space injection has a circumferential appearance.

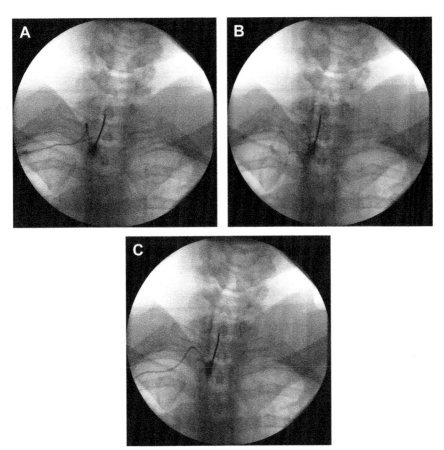

Fig. 11. Vascular contrast flow seen during a cervical interlaminar epidural injection AP view. (*A*) Precontrast. (*B*) Static image from live, real-time contrast injection demonstrating both epidural and vascular flow. (*C*) Image immediately following live injection. Note that live, real-time, dynamic fluoroscopic imaging (B) is needed to visualize the vascular flow. Otherwise, the vascular injection would have been missed.

epidural space (**Fig. 13**). Multiplanar views can be utilized to confirm that the contrast is in the facet joint. Medication localized to the facet joint is nonideal for an attempted epidural injection, and the needle should be repositioned to optimize epidural flow.

INTRADISCAL CONTRAST FLOW

Intradiscal contrast flow is a potential nonideal pattern seen with attempted transforaminal epidural injections (**Fig. 14**). This is particularly true with an infraneural (Kambin

Table 2
Distinguishing features between venous and arterial contrast flow

	Venous	Arterial
Pattern	Slower flow, often lateral and caudal	Rapid flow and wash out, often medial and cephalad
Inadvertent injection	Decreased efficacy	Decreased efficacy Potential stroke, spinal cord infarct

30

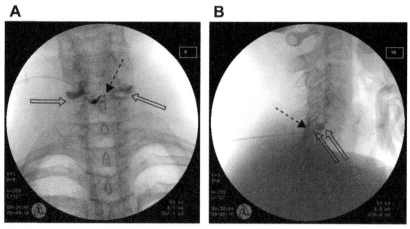

Fig. 12. Retrodural space of Okada injection. (*A*) AP view of a space of Okada injection during an attempted cervical interlaminar epidural injection with contrast flowing to the epidural space (*closed arrow*) and neighboring bilateral facet joints (open *arrows*). (*B*) Lateral view with both epidural (*closed arrow*) and facet joint (*open arrows*). (*Courtesy of* Justin Petrolla, MD, South Hills Orthopaedics surgery associates, Bethel park, PA; with permission.)

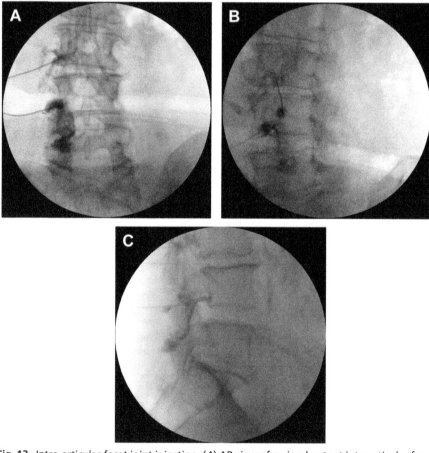

Fig. 13. Intra-articular facet joint injection. (*A*) AP view of an inadvertent intraarticular facet joint injection during an attempted left L4 transforaminal epidural injection (note, optimal epidural flow is seen at the L3 level). (*B*) Ipsilateral oblique view. (*C*) Lateral view. Note the vertical nature of the intra-articular facet joint contrast flow in all views.

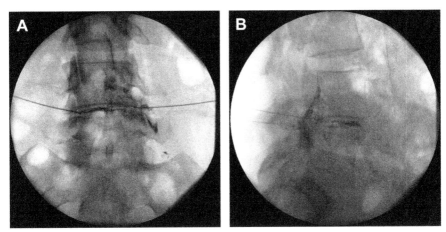

Fig. 14. Intradiscal injection. (*A*) AP view of an inadvertent intradiscal injection during an attempted left L4 transforaminal epidural injection via infraneural approach (note, the right-sided flow is optimal epidural flow). (*B*) Lateral view. Note the linear horizontal nature of flow on AP view and linear ventral flow on lateral view.

triangle) approach. Although using an infraneural approach has been suggested to decrease the likelihood of neural or vascular contact, it also increases the chances of penetrating the nearby disc, especially with herniated or bulging discs on the side of the attempted procedure. Intradiscal contrast flow has a linear, horizontal pattern localized to the disc space on AP view. Lateral view will demonstrate linear contrast flow moving ventrally in the intradiscal space. Medication localized to the disc space is nonideal for an attempted epidural injection, and the needle should be repositioned to optimize epidural flow.

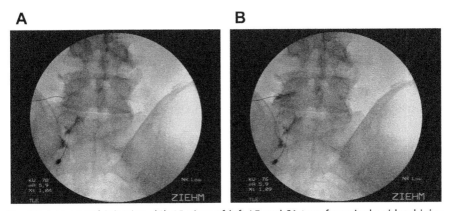

Fig. 15. Intraneural injection. (*A*) AP view of left L5 and S1 transforaminal epidural injections. Note that the L5 contrast flow pattern demonstrates a suboptimal train tracks contrast appearance after a painful intraneural injection. The train track appearance occurs for a similar reason discussed in **Fig. 7A**. The contrast outlines the dorsal root ganglion as well. Further injection before needle repositioning will be more painful and will potentially cause neural injury and is not recommended. (*B*) AP view of the same case after slightly pulling back on the L5 needle and confirming an epidural injection. Injectate was placed much more comfortably with this needle tip position.

| Box 1 |
| Differential for rapid contrast dilution |
| Rapid vascular uptake |
| Dilution effect (ie, intrathecal/subarachnoid) |
| Wrong syringe (no contrast) |

INTRANEURAL CONTRAST FLOW

During attempted transforaminal epidural injections, an intraneural injection can occur. The intraneural space is a potential space. Injection of contrast while in this location would cause significant discomfort to the patient and outline the periphery of the spinal nerve giving a train tracks pattern (see **Fig. 7**A; **Fig. 15**). Further injection before needle repositioning is not recommended, and often the needle should be slightly withdrawn for optimal needle placement in the epidural space.

DIFFERENTIAL FOR RAPID CONTRAST DILUTION

When injecting radio-opaque media, be aware of the differential for nonvisualized or minimally seen contrast (**Box 1**). Contrast taken up by venous or arterial structures should be seen with live standard fluoroscopy and enhanced with digital subtraction imaging. Contrast injected into the intrathecal/subarachnoid space is quickly diluted and not well visualized. Using pattern analysis described previously, this can be identified. Occasionally, a syringe may be mislabeled. It is best to note the contrast within the extension tubing under fluoroscopy as confirmation that the correct solution is in the syringe as well.

SUMMARY

Identifying and recognizing the significance of different contrast flow patterns are integral components of performing interventional spinal procedures. The practitioner should be aware of the distinct patterns discussed and be able to identify them and react accordingly. Recognizing a suboptimal contrast pattern with the potential for its potential complications is crucial to providing safe and effective procedures.

ACKNOWLEDGMENTS

Special thanks to Milton Landers, DO, and Tim Maus, MD, for their assistance in clarifying many of the concepts presented in this article.

REFERENCES

1. Lee SG, Choi SJ, Park MS, et al. Unexpected contrast filling during fluoroscopy guided epidural steroid injection; What should we do? Euorpean Soc Radiol 2015.
2. Neal J. Complications in regional anesthesia and pain medicine. Philadelphia (PA): Lippincott and Williams; 2013.
3. Furman MB, Jasper NR, Lin H. Fluoroscopic Contralateral Oblique View in Interlaminar Interventions: A technical note. Pain Medicine 2012;13(11):1389–96.
4. Goodman BS, Posecion LW, Mallempati S, et al. Complications and pitfalls of lumbar interlaminar and transforaminal epidural injections. Curr Rev Musculoskelet Med 2008;1(3–4):212–22.

5. Sadacharam K, Petersohn JD, Green MS. Inadvertent subdural injection during cervical transforaminal epidural steroid injection. Case Rep Anesthesiol 2013; 2013:1–5.
6. Levi D. Subdural extra-arachnoid flow pattern visualized in a contralateral oblique view during a cervical interlaminar epidural steroid injection. Pain Med 2017; 18(6):1177–82.
7. Furman MB, O'Brien EM, Zgleszewski TM. Incidence of intravascular penetration in transforaminal lumbosacral epidural steroid injections. Spine 2000;15:2628–32.
8. Furman MB, Giovanniello MT, O'Brien EM. Incidence of intravascular penetration in transforaminal cervical epidural steroid injections. Spine 2003;28:21–5.
9. Kim Y, Park H, Moon D. Rates of lumbosacral transforaminal injections interpreted as intravascular: Fluoroscopy alone or with digital subtraction. Anaesthesia 2013; 68:1120–3.
10. Visnjevac O, Kim P, Farid-Davari S, et al. Digital subtraction angiography versus realtime fluoroscopy for detection of intravascular penetration prior to epidural steroid injections: meta-analysis of prospective studies. Pain Physician 2015; 18:29–36.
11. Visnjevac O, Kim P, Farid-Davari S, et al. Digital Subtraction Angiography Versus Real Timee Fluoroscopy for Detection of Intravascular Penetration Prior to Epidural Steroid Injections: Meta-Analysis of Prospective Studies. Pain Physician 2015;18:29–36.
12. Murthy NS, Maus TP, Aprill C. The retrodural space of Okada. AJR Am J Roentgenol 2011;196(6):W784–9.

Lumbosacral Transitional Segments

An Interventional Spine Specialist's Practical Approach

Michael B. Furman, MD, MS[a,b,c],*, Brady Wahlberg, DO[a],
Eduardo J. Cruz, MD[d,e]

KEYWORDS

- Lumbosacral transitional vertebrae • Transitional segment anatomy • MRI
- Lumbarized S1 • Sacralized L5 • Radiculopathy • Spinal stenosis
- Herniated nucleus pulposis

KEY POINTS

- The presence of a lumbosacral transitional vertebra (LSTV) should prompt a more detailed preprocedural evaluation of the vertebral column to accurately determine spinal levels.
- An LSTV should prompt the use of corroborating intraprocedural imaging to verify morphology.
- The most important factors in treating lumbosacral transitional segments are communication among treating physicians to ensure segmental enumeration consistency and associated appropriate patient treatment.

INTRODUCTION

Lumbosacral transitional vertebrae (LTV) are congenital vertebral anomalies that may be present in up to 30% of the general population.[1] There is a wide variability range in transitional segment morphology from a broad transverse process up to complete fusion, which can be graded by the Castellvi classification.[2]

The authors have nothing to disclose.
[a] Interventional Spine and Sports Medicine Fellowship, OSS Health, 1855 Powder Mill Road, York, PA 17402, USA; [b] Special Consultant, Rehabilitation Medicine, Sinai Hospital of Baltimore, Baltimore, MD, USA; [c] Clinical Assistant Professor, Physical Medicine and Rehabilitation, Temple University School of Medicine, Philadelphia, PA, USA; [d] Spine & Sports, Ocala Family Medical Center, 2230 SW 19th Avenue Road, Ocala, FL 34471, USA; [e] Assistant Professor, Ocala Regional Medical Center, Ocala, FL, USA
* Corresponding author. Interventional Spine and Sports Medicine Fellowship, OSS Health, 1855 Powder Mill Road, York, PA 17402.
E-mail address: mbfurman@gmail.com

Phys Med Rehabil Clin N Am 29 (2018) 35–48
https://doi.org/10.1016/j.pmr.2017.08.004
1047-9651/18/© 2017 Elsevier Inc. All rights reserved.

pmr.theclinics.com

Lumbosacral transitional segments present a special challenge to the spine interventionalist. The fluoroscopic imaging makes level identification perplexing and final needle target/position unclear. Questions that typically arise in the procedure suite include: Is the transitional segment a lumbarized S1 or sacralized L5? What counting convention is the requesting physician using? Is it the same as the radiologist who read the imaging study? What are the clinical symptoms that the requesting physician wants us to treat when consulting for interventional procedures? What is the best way to count and identify the segments? Is there a sixth lumbar vertebra? Is using the iliac crest (IC) as a landmark for L4-L5 or counting from the thoracolumbar junction enough to correctly identify the vertebral level?

Treating or identifying the wrong level may be a major concern moving forward, because some of the patients that do not respond to conservative treatment may require surgery. Many options have been described to identify the transitional level (tl). These options include using anatomic landmarks on imaging, such as the iliolumbar ligament, renal artery, or IC, or using the MRI cervical scout images (when available) to count down from C2.

Each identification technique has its advantages; however, none of them provide 100% accuracy. Because correlating the tl to clinical presentation is crucial before performing any procedure, the authors share a logical, clinically oriented, approach to use before initiating a spinal procedure.

Lumbosacral vertebral anomalies and their clinical significance to back pain have been a topic of debate for years. There has not been a clear consensus on where exactly to treat, because patients with these anomalies may have pain generators that may be secondary to the motion segment above the transitional segment or contralateral facet arthropathy. Pain secondary to pseudoarthrosis formed by anatomic variation of the fifth lumbar vertebra has been reported as well. The anomalous fifth lumbar segment may articulate or fuse with the sacrum or IC. This articulation has been referred to Bertolotti syndrome and has been well described in the literature since 1917.

Although there has been uncertainty if transitional segments are a pain generator to consider in patients with back pain, a study by Nardo and colleagues[3,4] in 2012 demonstrated that LSTV types II and IV positively correlate with prevalence and severity of low back and buttock pain. There have been successful cases where this pseudoarthrosis has either been treated with local anesthetic/steroid or removed surgically.

Although the identification of these anatomic anomalies are challenging to identify, this article explores and emphasizes what is perceived to be the single most important factor in treating lumbosacral transitional segments: There must be unambiguous and concise communication among providers regarding the segmental enumeration convention utilized to assure consistency.

It has been reported that the most accurate method of identifying the lumbosacral transition is using anteroposterior (AP) and lateral lumbosacral radiographs combined with a 30° angled cranially directed AP plain (Ferguson) radiograph.[5–8] The lumbar levels can then be easily defined by counting down from the T12 vertebra, defined as the vertebra from which the lowest rib originates.[7] With this said, this does not allow identification of a thoracolumbar transitional vertebra or nontypical thoracolumbar segmental distribution, and an erroneous assumption is usually made of 12 thoracic segments. There is a possibility of extra or missing thoracic segments that may confuse the clinician when counting lumbosacral segments (see **Figs. 7–9**).

Some investigators regard computed tomography (CT) as the best imaging technique for characterization of LSTVs. These anomalies are usually identified incidentally because CT is not the preferred imaging technique used to evaluate patients with nontraumatic low back pain. In these clinical cases, MRI is more often indicated, given its superior tissue differentiation within and around the spine, and CT exposes the patient to radiation.[1]

With MRI alone, LSTVs can be detected either on coronal images, which highlight the transitional lumbosacral anatomy, or on axial images of the lumbosacral junction, which depict the pseudoarthrosis/fusion of the last lumbar vertebra with the sacrum. However, coronal images are not usually acquired in MRI examinations of the lumbar spine, whereas the lumbosacral junction may be erroneously identified at the L4-L5 level in sagittal scout images of subjects with LSTV. The images obtained may result in incomplete axial coverage of the transitional level and may be missed on MRI.[2] The classification and numbering of LSTVs are also problematic on MRI due to factors including limited imaging of the thoracolumbar junction, identification of the lowest rib-bearing vertebral body, and differentiation between thoracic hypoplastic ribs and enlarged lumbar transverse processes.[3]

Many techniques have been suggested to define the lumbar vertebral levels on MRIs. A consensus of determining the lumbosacral transition by radiological methods, nevertheless, is still lacking.[7,9–17]

Potential anatomic landmarks for vertebral labeling could be related to intrinsic spinal structures or paraspinal structures that are typically included in the field of view of routine lumbar spine MRI.[3] Nonspinal anatomic landmarks such as the abdominal vasculature are problematic because of their variable location and potential changes in location with age.[18] The use of intradural spinal landmarks, such as the conus medullaris or dural sac termination, can also be problematic because of their variable location in general. Although a study by Lee and colleagues[19] concluded that the aortic bifurcation, IC (inferior vena cava confluence), right renal artery, CT (celiac trunk), SR (superior mesenteric artery root), and iliolumbar ligament are useful landmarks for predicting the presence of LSTV on MRI, the aortic bifurcation and right renal artery are widely thought to be less than satisfactory.[11] Lee and colleagues[20] have also shown that the conus medullaris should not be used as a landmark because its position is quite variable. Unfortunately, as with other described landmarks, it has been shown that identification of the ILL (iliolumbar ligament) is not sufficiently accurate to denote the L5 vertebra.[3]

Prior reports of imaging investigations of LSTVs[9,10] advocate using total spine localizers for counting the total number of presacral segments. Radiographs of the entire spine allow for counting caudally from C2 and for differentiating hypoplastic ribs from lumbar transverse processes.[1]

Hahn and colleagues[9] first described the use of a sagittal cervicothoracic MR localizer to better evaluate transitional vertebrae. With a sagittal MR localizer, the vertebrae may be counted in a caudad direction from C2 rather than cephalad from L5. Using a sagittal cervicothoracic MR localizer alone assumes 7 cervical and 12 thoracic vertebrae and does not account for thoracolumbar transitions or allow differentiation of dysplastic ribs from lumbar transverse processes. The addition of a coronal MR cervicothoracic localizer increases the accuracy of enumerating LSTV[10] because it allows better differentiation at the thoracolumbar junction. However, given the large field of view and increased section thickness of these localizers, they still commonly do not provide enough reliable anatomic information to consistently number the segments of the lumbar spine correctly. In addition, many radiologists do not routinely obtain an MR localizer inclusive of the cervical and thoracic spine when imaging patients with low back pain, unless requested by the treating physicians.

Because no landmark is consistently reliable, making an explicit statement in the lumbar spine MRI report regarding how the lumbosacral junction was determined is advocated. If an LSTV is present, this should be stated along with its characterization, including where the lowest well-formed intervertebral disk is. This landmark can be identified at fluoroscopy during surgical or percutaneous procedures.[3]

Essentially without high-quality imaging of the entirety of the spine, there is no foolproof method for accurately numbering a transitional segment. Therefore, identification, communication with the referring clinician, and correlation of intraoperative and preoperative imaging become of paramount importance.[1] The presence of an LSTV should prompt preprocedural evaluation of the entire vertebral column to accurately determine spinal levels; in addition, an LSTV should prompt the use of corroborating intraprocedural imaging to verify morphology.

Innervation in the Setting of Transitional Segment Anatomy

Patients with a cranial displacement of the thoracolumbar or lumbosacral vertebral transition show a dermatome gap, which lies significantly more ventrally than in patients with a normal spinal configuration.[21] Findings in a study by Kim and colleagues[22] suggest that the function of the lumbosacral nerve roots is altered in patients with a sacralized L5, and that the L4 nerve root serves the usual function of the L5 nerve root. The altered function of the nerve roots support the notion of a variant position of lumbosacral dermatomes in the presence of transitional vertebrae, which manifests as poor correlation with clinical symptoms and may result in wrong levels for percutaneous injection procedures, which has significant clinical impact.

Hinterdorfer and colleagues[13] presented the first prospective comparative study estimating the innervation pattern of lumbar nerve roots in patients with 6 lumbar vertebral bodies (6LVB) using clinical signs and electrical stimulation via evoked EMG monitoring. Other clinicians may call the 6th lumbar vertebral body (6th LVB) a lumbarized S1 because there are no L6 innervated muscles or dermatomes described in the literature. Some studies have shown that L6 segments behave like S1 segments. The overall picture is that clinical pain distribution and the myotomal chart of electromyographically based patterns of muscle innervation in patients with 5 and in patients with 6LVB (lumbarized S1) showed that the presence of lumbarization does not significantly affect the segmental innervation. Thus, in general, patients matching the profile of 6LVB (lumbarized S1) may be diagnosed and treated in the same way as those with 5LVB.

Clinical Recommendations in the Setting of Transitional Segmentation

With no previous radiographs or MRIs available to allow the interventionalist to reach a decision for final needle target, obtaining a lateral view provides initial information.

Discussion and recommendations
With no or limited prior imaging: The patient is referred to the spine interventionalist for an evaluation and management.

1. Evaluate the patient and review all available imaging studies. If a transitional segment is suspected from plain spine films, obtain an MRI with a scout image for the purpose of counting caudad from C2 to the lumbosacral junction.

If available, identify the vertebral levels by counting down from the C2 vertebra using a scout midsagittal image on MRI.

2. Correlate identified abnormality from review of imaging studies with the radiologist's report and patient's clinical findings and then decide on a specific spine procedure.
3. During the procedure, correlate findings from previous imaging studies with the intraprocedural fluoroscopic images, plan the approach, accurately identify needle target, and perform the planned spine procedure.
4. Unambiguously document the enumeration convention used: lumbarized S1 versus sacralized L5. Include enumeration correlation with fluoroscopic images and any available imaged spine abnormality using the same consistent convention.

With no or limited prior imaging: The patient is referred to a spine interventionalist for a specific procedure.

1. The referring physician evaluates the patient and then orders a specific spine procedure based on the patient's signs and symptoms.
2. Evaluate the patient and correlate clinical findings with the ordered spine procedure. (At this point, you may decide to proceed with the ordered spine procedure or you may have to order and review any available spine imaging, talk to the referring physician, or change the ordered procedure depending on the clinical scenario, ie, appropriateness/urgency of the procedure, necessity of prior imaging, availability of imaging facilities, risks vs benefits of the procedure, and your relationship with the referring physician).
3. During the procedure, if there are no prior imaging studies and an LSTV is suspected from intraprocedural fluoroscopic images, obtain a fluoroscopic true AP image centered over the patient's lumbosacral junction. Pay special attention to the transverse processes of the lowest lumbar-appearing vertebra; take note of their size and whether either one or both are fused to the sacrum/ilium. Also take note of the lowest-appearing lumbar vertebrae's spatial relations to the IC.
4. Using the superior border of the IC as a landmark, obtain a fluoroscopic true lateral image centered over the lumbosacral junction. Correlate vertebral levels with pathologic findings.
5. Using the superior border of the ICs as a landmark, obtain a fluoroscopic true AP view centered over the lumbosacral junction. Correlate vertebral levels and pathologic findings with the fluoroscopic true lateral.
6. If doubt regarding vertebral levels persists, you may count down from the T12 vertebra, defined as the vertebra from which the lowest rib originates. Correlate levels identified with findings on AP, lateral and previous imaging studies (if available), and then plan the approach, accurately identify needle target, and perform the ordered/planned spine procedure.
7. Unambiguously document the enumeration convention used: Lumbarized S1 versus sacralized L5. Include enumeration correlation with the referring physician's ordered procedure, the fluoroscopic images, and any available imaged spine abnormality using the same consistent convention.

With prior imaging: The patient is referred to the spine interventionalist for an evaluation and management.

1. Evaluate the patient, review prior imaging studies, and decide on a specific spine procedure. If a transitional segment is suspected from review of prior imaging

studies and an MRI is to be ordered, an MRI scout image is recommended for the purpose of counting caudad from C2 to the lumbosacral junction. If available, identify the vertebral levels by counting down from the C2 vertebra using a scout midsagittal image on MRI.

2. Correlate identified abnormality from review of imaging studies with the radiologist's report and patient's clinical findings and then decide on a specific spine procedure and identify needle target.
3. During the procedure, correlate findings from previous imaging studies (a scout midsagittal image on MRI) with the intraprocedural fluoroscopic images, plan the approach, accurately identify needle target, and perform the planned spine procedure.
4. Unambiguously document the enumeration convention used: Lumbarized S1 versus sacralized L5. Include enumeration correlation with the interpreting radiologist's enumeration, the fluoroscopic images, and any available imaged spine abnormality using the same consistent convention.

With prior imaging: The patient is referred to the spine interventionalist for a specific procedure.

1. The referring physician evaluates the patient, orders, reviews, and interprets imaging studies and then orders a specific spine procedure.
2. Evaluate the patient, review the patient's records including prior imaging studies, and correlate with the ordered spine procedure. (At this point, you may decide to proceed with the ordered spine procedure or you may have to order and review other spine imaging, talk to the referring physician, or change the ordered procedure depending on the clinical scenario, ie, appropriateness/urgency of the procedure, necessity of other imaging, availability of imaging facilities, risks vs benefits of the procedure, and your relationship with the referring physician).
3. If a transitional segment is suspected from review of prior imaging studies and an MRI is to be ordered, an MRI scout image is recommended for the purpose of counting caudad from C2 to the lumbosacral junction. If available, identify the vertebral levels by counting down from the C2 vertebra using a scout midsagittal image on MRI.
4. Correlate identified abnormality from review of imaging studies with the radiologist's report and patient's clinical findings.
5. During the procedure, correlate identified abnormality from review of imaging studies (a scout midsagittal image on MRI) with the radiologist's report, referring physician's interpretation of prior imaging studies, and patient's clinical findings with the intraprocedural fluoroscopic images, plan the approach, accurately identify needle target, and perform the ordered/planned spine procedure.
6. Unambiguously document the enumeration convention used: lumbarized S1 versus sacralized L5. Include enumeration correlation with the interpreting radiologist's enumeration, the referring physician's ordered procedure, the fluoroscopic images, and any available imaged spine abnormality using the same consistent convention.

In order to accurately and consistently correlate vertebral levels and abnormality with treatment, there needs to be consistency and accuracy of identification and communication of the vertebral levels among clinicians. It is most important to correlate the patient's clinical symptoms with the pathoanatomy visualized on the imaging that is obtained. Subsequently, images obtained during the procedure need to be correlated with the same visualized pathoanatomy.

In summary, identifying and consistently enumerating transitional anatomy are critical before a surgical or percutaneous procedure to avoid wrong-level exposure or injection. Communication between providers will ensure consistency. The use of intraoperative imaging is promoted[23,24] to avoid mistakes of wrong-level procedures. Because the presence of an LSTV makes it about 7 times more likely that an individual has an anomalous number of presacral vertebrae, identification of an LSTV should prompt additional imaging for verifying numbering, particularly if an intervention is contemplated, to reduce the ambiguity that the presence of an LSTV might introduce.

Lumbosacral Transitional Segmentation Examples

Example 1: Bilateral L5 transforaminal epidural steroid injection performed in a patient with a lumbarized S1 transitional segment (**Figs. 1–3**)

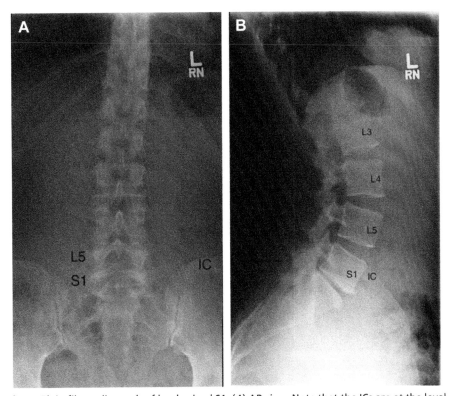

Fig. 1. Plain film radiograph of lumbarized S1. (*A*) AP view. Note that the ICs are at the level of the superior endplate of the lumbarized S1. (*B*) Lateral view. Note that the IC is at the level of the superior endplate of the lumbarized S1.

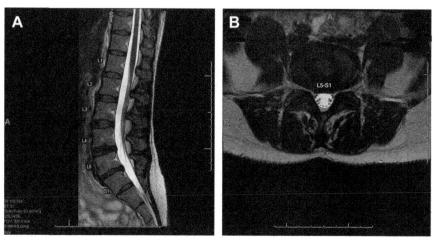

Fig. 2. T2-weighted MRI lumbarized S1. (This is the same patient as in **Fig. 1.**) (*A*) Sagittal with the vertebral bodies labeled. The L5-S1 level is the last fully formed disc space. There is evidence of a rudimentary S1-S2 disc. (*B*) Axial view through L5-S1 disc.

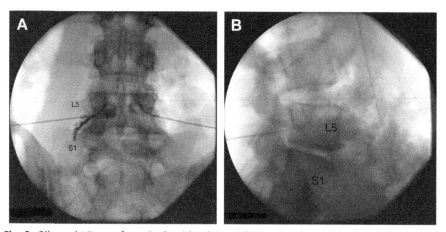

Fig. 3. Bilateral L5 transforaminal epidural steroid injections in a patient with lumbarized S1. (This is the same patient as in **Figs. 1** and **2**.) Comparing preprocedure plain film radiographs (see **Fig. 1**) and MRI (see **Fig. 2**), the interventionalist can perform bilateral L5 transforaminal injections. (*A*) AP fluoroscopy demonstrates that the ICs are at the superior border of S1. (*B*) Lateral fluoroscopy demonstrates that the IC is at the level of the superior endplate of S1. L5-S1 is the last fully formed disc. The rudimentary S1-S2 space is visualized, and the appropriate level of needle placement is able to be confirmed.

Example 2: Left L4 and L5 transforaminal epidural steroid injection performed in a patient with a sacralized L5 transitional segment (**Figs. 4–6**)

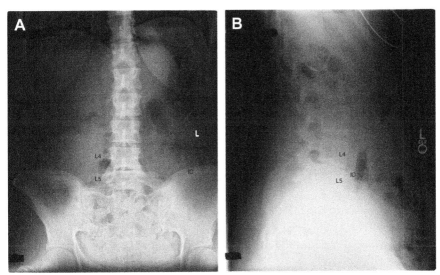

Fig. 4. Plain film radiograph sacralized L5. (*A*) AP view. Note that the ICs are at the level of the superior endplate of the sacralized L5. (*B*) Lateral. Although the sacral segments are not well visualized, one can still appreciate that the ICs are at the level of L4-L5.

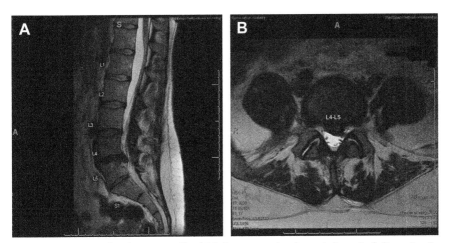

Fig. 5. (*A, B*) T2-weighted MRI sacralized L5 demonstrating large left central disc extrusion at L4-L5. (This is the same patient as in **Figs. 4** and **6**.)

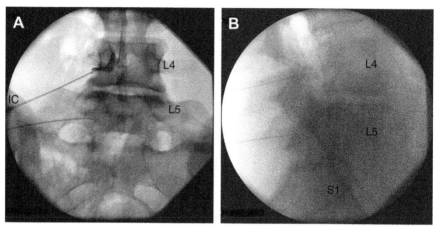

Fig. 6. (*A*) AP fluoroscopy demonstrating left L4 and L5 transforaminal epidural needle placement in a patient with sacralized L5 with known large left disc extrusion at L4-L5. Note the IC is at the level of the superior endplate of L5. (This is the same patient as in **Figs. 4** and **5**.) (*B*) Lateral fluoroscopy demonstrating left L4 and L5 transforaminal epidural needle placement in a patient with sacralized L5.

Example 3: T12-L1 percutaneous disc biopsy performed in a patient with 6 non-rib-bearing vertebrae (**Figs. 7–9**)

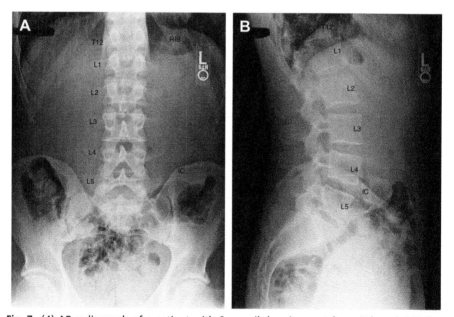

Fig. 7. (*A*) AP radiograph of a patient with 6 non-rib-bearing vertebrae. Where is L5? One way to label the anatomy of this patient is to declare the ICs at the "L5-L6" level. Another possible label is to declare that the last space is the L5-S1 space. The nomenclature cannot be named without a scout midsagittal MRI with counting caudad from C2 to the lumbosacral junction. The plain film above is labeled according to the radiologist's count in the lumbar MRI in **Fig. 8**A, B. (*B*) Lateral radiograph of a patient with 6 non-rib-bearing vertebrae. (This is the same patient in **Fig. 7**A.) The plain film above is labeled according to the radiologist's count in the lumbar MRI in **Fig. 8**A, B.

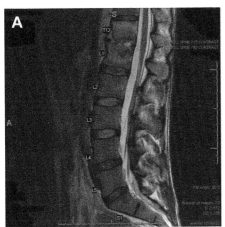
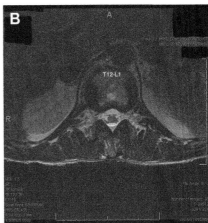

Fig. 8. (A, B) T2-weighted MRI demonstrating findings suspicious for discitis/osteomyelitis at T12-L1 in a patient with an atypical count. (This is the same patient as in Fig. 7.) Note the radiologist called the last disc space the L5-S1 level. The T12-L1 level was identified counting in a cephalad direction, starting at the most caudal fully formed disc space. In this case, a scout MRI image was not available. For practical purposes, the most important point to note is that when performing the procedure, the interventionalist must count L5-S1 as the last space. The T12-L1 level was not determined by counting caudally from the ribs. Grade I retrolisthesis of T12 in respect to L1 is also visualized.

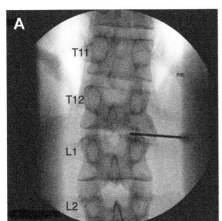
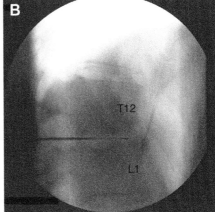

Fig. 9. (A) AP fluoroscopy of T12-L1 percutaneous disc biopsy. Note that if the T12-L1 would have been identified by counting in a caudad direction starting at the ribs, the incorrect disc would have been accessed. (B) Lateral fluoroscopy of T12-L1 percutaneous disc biopsy. Note the T12-L1 is also confirmed in the lateral view by visualizing known grade I retrolisthesis of T12 with respect to L1 that was seen on prior imaging for comparison.

Example 4: Left L4 and L5 transforaminal epidural steroid injection performed in a patient with 6 lumbar vertebrae in the setting of a discrepancy of labeling of the vertebral bodies between the ordering physician of the procedure and the radiologist. (In this case, the nomenclature refers to the labeling from each physician in this particular case. This does not refer to a standard of labeling used by all radiologists and spine surgeons; **Figs. 10–12.**)

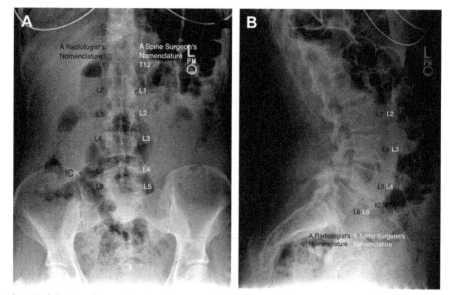

Fig. 10. (*A*) AP radiograph: 6 lumbar vertebrae. Where is L5? One way to label the anatomy of this patient is to declare the ICs at the "L5-L6" level. Another possible label is to declare that the last space is the L5-S1 space. The nomenclature cannot be named without a scout midsagittal MRI image with counting caudad from C2 to the lumbosacral junction. In this particular case, a spine surgeon and a radiologist labeled the lumbar vertebrae differently. (*B*) Lateral radiograph demonstrating anterolisthesis of L5 on "L6" in a patient with 6 lumbar vertebrae, according to the radiologist's read of the study. The spine surgeon who ordered the procedure declared that the patient had anterolisthesis of L4 on L5. Note the discrepancies between the 2 physicians.

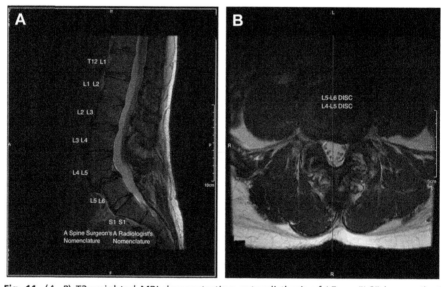

Fig. 11. (*A, B*) T2-weighted MRI demonstrating anterolisthesis of L5 on "L6" in a patient with 6 lumbar vertebrae, according to the radiologist. T2-weighted MRI demonstrating anterolisthesis of L4 on L5, according to a spine surgeon. In this example, the radiologist noted 6 lumbar-type vertebrae in the MRI report, with the last space called the "L6-S1" disc space. A spine surgeon ordered a left L4 and L5 transforaminal epidural steroid injection. A closer look at the spine surgeon's note revealed a dictation of a grade II anterolisthesis of L4 on L5, and a left L4 and L5 transforaminal epidural steroid injection was ordered to target the disc protrusion above and below the level of the anterolisthesis.

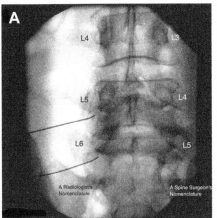
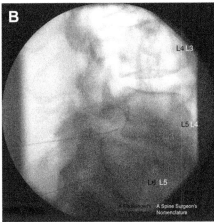

Fig. 12. (*A*) AP fluoroscopy of left L4 and L5 transforaminal epidural needle placement in a patient with 6 lumbar vertebrae when ordering physician-called anterolisthesis of L4 on L5. (*B*) Lateral fluoroscopy of left L4 and L5 transforaminal epidural needle placement in a patient with 6 lumbar vertebrae when ordering physician-called anterolisthesis of L4 on L5. Note that the interventionalist can confirm that in the lateral view that a 2-level transforaminal injection was performed above and below the area of the anterolisthesis.

SUMMARY

Essentially without high-quality imaging of the entirety of the spine including a scout, there is no foolproof method for accurately numbering a transitional segment; therefore, identification, communication with the referring clinician, and correlation of preprocedural and intraprocedural imaging become of paramount importance.[1] Therefore, the presence of an LSTV should prompt a more detailed preprocedural evaluation of the vertebral column to accurately determine spinal levels; in addition, an LSTV should prompt the use of corroborating intraprocedural imaging to verify morphology. The authors submit that the most important factors in treating lumbosacral transitional segments is communication among treating physicians to ensure segmental enumeration consistency and associated appropriate patient treatment.

REFERENCES

1. Konin GP, Walz DM. Lumbosacral transitional vertebrae: classification, imaging findings, and clinical relevance. AJNR Am J Neuroradiol 2010;31:1778–86.
2. Chalian M, Soldatos T, Carrino JA, et al. Prediction of transitional lumbosacral anatomy on magnetic resonance imaging of the lumbar spine. World J Radiol 2012;4(3):97–101.
3. Nardo L, Alizai H, Virayavanich W, et al. Lumbosacral transitional vertebrae: association with low back pain. Radiology 2012;265(2):497–503.
4. Wigh RE. The thoracolumbar and lumbosacral transitional junctions. Spine (Phila Pa 1976) 1980;5(3):215–22.
5. Cimen M, Elden H. Numerical variations in human vertebral column: a case report. Okajimas Folia Anat Jpn 1999;75:297–303.
6. Ebraheim NA, Xu R. Assessment of lumbosacral fusion mass by angled radiography. Technical notes. Spine 1998;23:842–3.

7. Hughes RJ, Saifuddin A. Imaging of lumbosacral transitional vertebrae. Clin Radiol 2004;59:984–91.
8. Tini PG, Wieser C, Zinn WM. The transitional vertebra of the lumbosacral spine: its radiological classification, incidence, prevalence, and clinical significance. Rheumatol Rehabil 1977;16:180–5.
9. Hahn PY, Strobel JJ, Hahn FJ. Verification of lumbosacral segments on MR images: identification of transitional vertebrae. Radiology 1992;182(2):580–1.
10. Peh WC, Siu TH, Chan JH. Determining the lumbar vertebral segments on magnetic resonance imaging. Spine (Phila Pa 1976) 1999;24(17):1852–5.
11. Hughes RJ, Saifuddin A. Numbering of lumbosacral transitional vertebrae on MRI: role of the iliolumbar ligaments. AJR Am J Roentgenol 2006;187:W59–65.
12. Bron JL, van Royen BJ, Wuisman PI. The clinical significance of lumbosacral transitional anomalies. Acta Orthop Belg 2007;73:687–95.
13. Hinterdorfer P, Parsaei B, Stieglbauer K, et al. Segmental innervation in lumbosacral transitional vertebrae (LSTV): a comparative clinical and intraoperative EMG study. J Neurol Neurosurg Psychiatry 2010;81(7):734–41.
14. Chithriki M, Jaibaji M, Steele RD. The anatomical relationship of the aortic bifurcation to the lumbar vertebrae: a MRI study. Surg Radiol Anat 2002;24:308–12.
15. Desmond PM, Buirski G. Magnetic resonance appearances of developmental disc anomalies in the lumbar spine. Australas Radiol 1993;37:26–9.
16. O'Driscoll CM, Irwin A, Saifuddin A. Variations in morphology of the lumbosacral junction on sagittal MRI: correlation with plain radiography. Skeletal Radiol 1996;25:225–30.
17. Ralston MD, Dykes TA, Applebaum BI. Verification of lumbar vertebral bodies. Radiology 1992;185:615–6.
18. Kornreich L, Hadar H, Sulkes J, et al. Effect of normal ageing on the sites of aortic bifurcation and inferior vena cava confluence: a CT study. Surg Radiol Anat 1998;20(1):63–8.
19. Lee CH, Park CM, Kim KA, et al. Identification and prediction of transitional vertebrae on imaging studies: anatomical significance of paraspinal structures. Clin Anat 2007;20:905–14.
20. Lee CH, Seo BK, Choi CY, et al. Using MRI to evaluate anatomic significance of aortic bifurcation, right renal artery, and conus medullaris when locating lumbar vertebral segments. AJR Am J Roentgenol 2004;182:1295–300.
21. Seyfert S. Dermatome variations in patients with transitional vertebrae. J Neurol Neurosurg Psychiatry 1997;63(6):801–3.
22. Kim YH, Lee PB, Lee CJ, et al. Dermatome variation of lumbosacral nerve roots in patients with transitional lumbosacral vertebrae. Anesth Analg 2008;106(4):1279–83.
23. Ammerman JM, Ammerman MD, Dambrosia J, et al. A prospective evaluation of the role for intraoperative x-ray in lumbar discectomy: predictors of incorrect level exposure. Surg Neurol 2006;66(5):470–3 [discussion: 473–4].
24. Mody MG, Nourbakhsh A, Stahl DL, et al. The prevalence of wrong level surgery among spine surgeons. Spine (Phila Pa 1976) 2008;33(2):194–8.

Ultrasound for Lumbar Spinal Procedures

Michelle Chi, MD[a], Allen S. Chen, MD, MPH[b],*

KEYWORDS

- Ultrasound • Ultrasonography • Interventional spine • Interventional pain
- Spine injections • Epidural • Facet • Medial branch block

KEY POINTS

- Ultrasound-guided spine interventions are becoming more frequently used.
- Ultrasound guidance can be used for several spine procedures, including facet injections, medial branch blocks, epidural injections, and sacroiliac joint injections.
- Advantages and disadvantages should be weighed carefully when deciding between ultrasound and other methods of visualization, such as fluoroscopy and computed tomography (CT).
- Interventionalists should be aware of limitations of ultrasound, particularly when spinal vasculature may be at risk.
- Further studies are needed to further evaluate safety and efficacy of ultrasound-guided procedures in comparison to fluoroscopy and CT.

INTRODUCTION

Image-guided injection techniques are an integral part of multimodal pain management, and ultrasonography has become an increasingly valuable and promising tool for performing these procedures. The increase in the use of ultrasound guidance has led to an increasing interest in the study of ultrasound-guided interventional spine procedures. Several studies have investigated the novel use of ultrasound for lumbosacral pain management procedures with favorable outcomes.

The successful practice of ultrasound-guided injections requires a thorough understanding of basic ultrasound principles and lumbosacral spine sonoanatomy. Several other key factors include appropriate identification of bone, soft tissue, and neural

The authors have nothing to disclose.
[a] Department of Rehabilitation and Regenerative Medicine, New York Presbyterian Hospital of Columbia and Cornell, Harkness Pavilion, 180 Fort Washington Avenue, St 1-199, New York, NY 10032, USA; [b] Department of Rehabilitation and Regenerative Medicine, Columbia University Medical Center, Harkness Pavillion, 180 Fort Washington Avenue, St 1-199, New York, NY 10032, USA
* Corresponding author.
E-mail address: asc2206@cumc.columbia.edu

Phys Med Rehabil Clin N Am 29 (2018) 49–60
https://doi.org/10.1016/j.pmr.2017.08.005
1047-9651/18/© 2017 Elsevier Inc. All rights reserved.

structures, defining essential ultrasound views, and successfully tracking the needle in real time. This article provides an overview of ultrasound-guided spine procedures and review of literature describing the methodology and feasibility of sonography for various lumbar spine injections, including medial branch blocks (MBBs), facet joint injections, epidural steroid injections, and sacroiliac (SI) joint injections.

BASIC ULTRASOUND PRINCIPLES

An ultrasound beam is generated when multiple piezoelectric crystals positioned along the surface of the transducer rapidly vibrate, creating an electrical field.[1] The sound waves that are produced are then reflected, refracted, and scattered while penetrating tissues of various acoustic impedance.[1] An image is subsequently displayed when some of the mechanical or sound energy that is returned to the transducer is converted into electrical energy.[1,2] Objects that appear lighter are termed "hyperechoic" and indicate higher signal intensity, whereas objects that appear darker are termed "hypoechoic" and indicate lower signal intensity.

Image quality is dependent on the angle of the ultrasound beam and is best when perpendicular to the target. High-frequency ultrasound is also associated with better resolution but varies inversely with depth of tissue penetration.[2] There are 2 scanning approaches used when performing ultrasound-guided injections: (1) The in-plane approach allows for complete visualization of the needle during its trajectory, but may be more challenging because the beam must be accurately aligned with the needle. (2) The out-of-plane approach depicts the needle as a bright dot, which may be difficult to localize and does not produce an image of the needle in its entirety.

LUMBOSACRAL SONOANATOMY

A low-frequency curved array transducer (2–6 MHz) is commonly used to visualize the lumbosacral spine and its neuraxial structures with depths that range from 5 to 7 cm. Bony structures that are identifiable with ultrasonography include spinous processes, transverse processes, vertebral laminae, articular processes, facet joints, and the posterior aspect of the vertebral bodies. Soft tissue structures, such as lumbar nerve roots, paraspinal muscles, ligamentum flavum, and posterior dura can also be visualized.[3]

Many lumbar procedures begin with a long-axis view to determine appropriate spinal levels. Then, the transducer is translated to the affected side to visualize lamina, facet joints, and transverse processes (**Fig. 1**). Once appropriate targets and levels

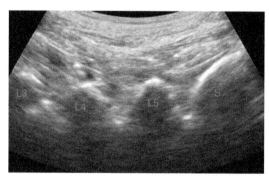

Fig. 1. Paramedian longitudinal view, lumbar spine. Lamina appear as a sawtooth pattern: (*left*) cranial; (*right*) caudal. S, sacrum. (*Courtesy of* Allen S. Chen, MD, MPH, New York, NY.)

are identified in the long-axis view, the probe is rotated to view structures in an axial plane, or transverse view.

Three important transverse views are often used during ultrasound-guided spine injections. The transverse spinous process view allows for visualization of the lamina, superior articular process (SAP), and transverse process (**Fig. 2**). The visibility of the facet joints, transverse processes, and SAPs in the transverse spinous process view is particularly useful when performing lumbar MBBs.

In the transverse interlaminar view, the vertebral canal and its associated structures can be seen, and in the transverse oblique foraminal view, the neuroforamen and lumbar paraspinals can be identified.[3]

ULTRASOUND ADVANTAGES AND LIMITATIONS

The rising trend in the use of ultrasonography for interventional lumbar spine procedures is attributable to its unique advantages over other imaging modalities (ie, computed tomography [CT], fluoroscopy). These modalities include avoidance of radiation exposure, real-time needle tracking from skin puncture to target, reduced equipment expenses, portability, and potentially reduction in block-related complications.[3]

However, some limitations also exist, largely because of ultrasound mechanics. Deeper structures within the lumbar spine, including the epidural space, dura, and spinal cord, may be difficult to identify because of obscurement from high acoustic impedance (ie, bony artifacts).[3,4] In addition, clear detection of intravascular injection is often difficult in comparison to CT and fluoroscopy.[3,4] Several other factors can affect the quality of an ultrasound image and impair needle visualization. Anatomic constraints, such as body habitus, bone hyperplasia, and degenerative changes can further reduce the ability to clearly delineate anatomic landmarks.[3] Echointensity of muscles also increase with age, often making visualization difficult.[5] Given these constraints, additional clinical research investigating the accuracy and safety of ultrasound-guided spinal injections over other standard image-guided modalities warrants further investigation.

LUMBAR FACET MEDIAL BRANCH BLOCKS

Lumbar facet pain is a common cause of chronic low back pain, with prevalence rates that increase with age, ranging from 15% to 45%.[3] Facet-mediated pain can arise from several structures associated with the facet joints (fibrous capsule, synovial

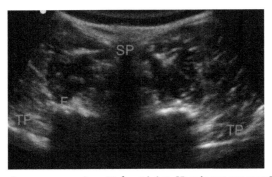

Fig. 2. Transverse spinous process view. FJ, facet joint; SP, spinous process; TP, transverse process. (*Courtesy of* Edward Pang, DO, Los Angeles, CA.)

membrane, hyaline cartilage, bone).[4] The currently accepted standard for diagnosing facet joint–mediated pain is through a series of facet nerve blocks, also referred to as medial branch blocks (MBBs). The medial branch of the dorsal primary ramus primarily innervates the facet joint. The lumbar dorsal ramus divides into medial, lateral, and intermediate branches approximately 5 mm from the proximal origin.[6] The medial branch lies in groove at the base of the SAP where it crosses the transverse process.[6,7]

Several cadaver and clinical studies have evaluated the efficacy and feasibility of ultrasound-guided MBBs. Defining sonographic landmarks and obtaining necessary ultrasound views are important for performing safe and accurate ultrasound-guided lumbar spine procedures. In 2004, Greher and colleagues[6,7] introduced a methodologic approach for performing ultrasound-guided lumbar medial branch blocks. The target point for the MBB lies on the upper margin of the transverse process and in the groove at the base of the SAP, where the medial branch traverses upper edge of the transverse process in a position ventrocranial to the mamilloaccessory ligament.

Technique

As with fluoroscopically guided procedures, the optimal positioning for injection purposes is with the patient prone with a pillow placed under the abdomen to reduce lumbar lordosis. A systematic approach is then used for detecting essential anatomic landmarks for target needle placement. First, the transverse process of the lumbar vertebrae is identified in longitudinal or long-axis view by counting from sacrum upward.[6,7] This long-axis view is used initially to determine appropriate target levels. The transducer is then rotated 90° into transverse view to delineate the step-off between the transverse process and SAP of the adjacent facet joint (**Fig. 3**).

After optimal visualization, a spinal needle is inserted laterally from the midline at an angle 45° to 60° to the skin. It is then advanced from lateral to medial until the needle tip reaches the junction between the SAP and superior border of the transverse process.[6,7] The needle should be visible in view while it is advanced toward the groove. Once bony contact is felt, the transducer is rotated back to longitudinal view to confirm position of the needle tip at the cranial edge of the transverse process.[6,7] Once the needle tip location is confirmed, local anesthetic is injected.

Greher and colleagues[6,7] studied the above described approach in 20 healthy volunteers using a 3.5-MHz curved array transducer at levels L3-L5. Various sonographic distances were measured, including the vertical distance (depth) from the skin to the

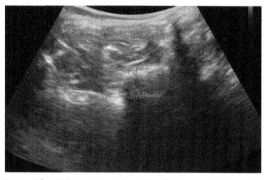

Fig. 3. Transverse view with MBB target at junction between SAP and TP. FJ, facet joint; SP, spinous process. (*Courtesy of* Allen S. Chen, MD, MPH, New York, NY.)

target point, and the lateral distance, from midline to the target.[6,7] Final needle placement was confirmed by C-arm fluoroscopy according to the current International Spine Intervention Society guidelines: slightly medial to the lateral margin of the SAP in the posteroanterior view, and "high on the eye of the Scottie dog" in oblique view.[6–8] The results of this study showed correct placement of all needles in their cadaver study, and all but 1 subject with a body mass index (BMI) of 36 showed successful identification of the appropriate landmarks.[6,7] A subsequent study by Greher and colleagues[7] was conducted to assess the accuracy and validity of the previously described approach using CT scan controls. Axial transverse CT scans with contrast were performed following needle placement, and spread of contrast medium was observed, with a success rate of 94%. These findings provided early evidence of the use of ultrasound as a promising guidance technique for lumbar spine MBBs.

Subsequent trials evaluating the efficacy of ultrasound-guided MBBs have also been published. Shim and colleagues[8] conducted a study of 20 patients and 101 MBBs confirmed with fluoroscopy and contrast.[8] The target point was defined as the groove of the cephalad margin of the transverse process adjacent to the SAP.[8] A 21-gauge spinal needle was introduced using in-plane approach to reach the target point. Then, 0.2 mL of contrast was injected and followed by fluoroscopy for confirmation of position.[8] Shim's study showed a successful needle placement rate of 95%.[8] This study illustrated that blocks were possible as long as the SAP and transverse process were both visible.[8]

L5 Dorsal Ramus Block

The L5-S1 facet joint, which is innervated by the L4 MBB and L5 dorsal ramus, is one of the most commonly affected joints in the spine.[9] However, given the surrounding anatomic structures, performing an L5 dorsal ramus block under ultrasound can be more challenging. The proximity of the iliac crest and the prominent lateral sacral crest makes visualization of the target more difficult than at other lumbar levels.

Greher and colleagues[9] described an approach for performing an L5 dorsal ramus block under ultrasound. With the ultrasound in a paramedian sagittal transverse process view, the sacrum can be visualized as a continuous hyperechogenic line caudal to the L5 transverse process. The transducer is then rotated in a partially oblique fashion, with visualization of iliac crest and sacral ala. The target is located at the sacral ala at the transition to the SAP (**Fig. 4**). The needle is then inserted in an oblique out-of-plane approach from a craniolateral to caudomedial position until bony contact

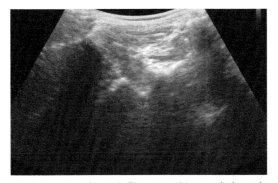

Fig. 4. L5 dorsal ramus transverse view. IC, iliac crest; SA, sacral ala and target for L5 dorsal ramus block. (*Courtesy of* Allen S. Chen, MD, MPH, New York, NY.)

is achieved. The transducer is then rotated back to sagittal transverse process view for confirmation of needle placement.[9]

In Greher's study, 20 ultrasound-guided L5 dorsal ramus blocks in 10 cadavers were performed with an 80% success rate.[9] Although these findings further support that the above described approach may be a feasible method for performing ultrasound-guided L5 dorsal ramus blocks, further studies evaluating the accuracy and efficacy in a clinical setting are needed.

LUMBAR FACET JOINT INTRA-ARTICULAR INJECTIONS

When performing facet joint injections, a similar systematic approach used for MBBs is also used to identify the target joint space, which has been defined as the midpoint or center of the cephalad-caudal extension of the lumbar facet joint space.[10]

Technique

The current literature describes several methods for obtaining optimal needle positioning and views for a successful facet joint injection. As with other spine procedures, the appropriate spinal level should first be defined in the long-axis view. The transducer is then rotated to a transverse view and moved along the spinous process until the lower margin of the lamina is delineated.[10] When the transducer is traced along the margin of the lamina to the lateral and caudal aspect, the inferior articular process of the joint with its medial facet can be seen, and the next occurring space encountered is the joint space.[10] In cases where the joint space is unclear, the area just medial to the SAP can alternatively be selected as the target[11] (**Fig. 5**). Once adequate views are achieved, the needle is inserted 3 to 4 cm laterally from the midline in a transverse plane at an angle of approximately 45° until the target is reached.[10] Although intra-articular placement is ideal, it is not always necessary for obtaining an appropriate spread of injectate. A subcapsular injection into the posterior synovial recess has also been shown to be effective and may reduce risk of damage to the joint cartilage.[11]

Several studies evaluating the feasibility and accuracy of using an ultrasound-guided approach for facet joint injections in the lumbar spine have been described. An earlier cadaver study by Galiano and colleagues[10] compared various measurements taken from a reference point using ultrasound and CT and assessed the differences between both imaging modalities. The results showed same mean measurements for both modalities. In a subsequent randomized controlled trial comparing ultrasound-guided versus CT-controlled facet joint injections, 40 adults with chronic low back pain were randomized to the CT or ultrasound-guided

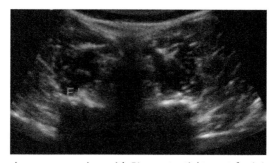

Fig. 5. Transverse spinous process view with FJ as potential target for injection. (*Courtesy of* Edward Pang, DO, Los Angeles, CA.)

group.[10,12] Outcome measures included procedure duration, radiation dose, and pain reduction using the visual analogue scale (VAS). All subjects received a mixture of 3 mL containing 1 mL 1% lidocaine, 1 mL 0.5% bupivacaine, and 1 mL (4 mg) beta-methasone. The ultrasound group was found to have a significant reduction in procedure duration and radiation dose compared with the CT group, demonstrating the use of ultrasound guidance for facet joints as a promising intervention.[12]

A later preclinical experiment compared ultrasound-guided facet joint injections with fluoroscopy control in cadavers.[11] This study was the first to use contrast injection to observe spread. After the target landmark was identified, 0.2 to 0.3 mL contrast was injected and followed by anteroposterior and oblique fluoroscopic views. The results showed an 88% success rate of having clear intra-articular contrast spread, further supporting the feasibility and efficacy of ultrasound-guided facet injections.[11]

Some limitations to this technique also exist. BMI plays an important role in the ability to visualize lumbar facet joints. In some studies, those with higher BMIs were not appropriate candidates due to the difficulty obtaining clear visualization of the facet joints.[12] Therefore, ultrasound-guided facet joint injections may be most effective for a select group of patients with normal BMIs.[4,12]

CAUDAL EPIDURAL INJECTIONS

Park and colleagues[13] investigated the feasibility and accuracy of ultrasound-guided caudal epidural steroid injections in a prospective randomized single-blind study comparing ultrasound with fluoroscopic guidance. In this approach, the ultrasound transducer is first placed in midline short-axis view, with visualization of the 2 sacral cornua, sacrococcygeal ligament, and sacral hiatus. The sacral cornua is observed as 2 hyperechoic structures forming an upside down "U". The sacrococcygeal ligament is seen as the superior of 2 hyperechoic bandlike structures in between the sacral cornua, with the sacral surface as the inferior band. The hypoechoic region between these 2 structures is the sacral hiatus (**Fig. 6**). Once these structures are delineated, a spinal needle is directed in between the 2 cornua and into the sacral hiatus. Once the sacrococcygeal ligament is penetrated, the transducer is rotated into longitudinal view and the needle is advanced into the sacral canal. After final needle placement, 1 to 2 cc of contrast is injected, and using color Doppler mode, flow is observed. A positive flow is indicated by unidirectional movement of contrast through the epidural space in 1 dominant color.[13]

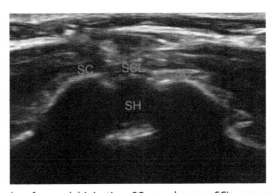

Fig. 6. Transverse view for caudal injection. SC, sacral cornu; SCL, sacrococcygeal ligament; SH, sacral hiatus. (*Courtesy of* Allen S. Chen, MD, MPH, New York, NY.)

In Park's randomized study, 120 patients with unilateral radicular pain were randomized to either the fluoroscopic or ultrasound group. In both groups, 5 cc of contrast and 15 cc of a mixed solution containing 0.5% lidocaine and 2 cc dexamethasone 10 mg were injected. Pertinent findings include shorter procedure duration in the ultrasound group and similar improvements in pain relief and function.[13] Park and colleagues[14] later evaluated the long-term effects of ultrasound-guided caudal epidural steroid injections compared with fluoroscopic control in a retrospective comparative study and found that both groups showed significant improvements in various parameters including the Oswestry Disability Index and VAS at the end of a 1-year period.

One potential advantage to using ultrasound for caudal epidural steroid injections is that it provides clearer images of the sacral hiatus and therefore may easier to perform in patients with more complex anatomic variations. However, visualizing Doppler flow can be challenging and may be difficult to distinguish epidural flow from vascular flow. Another disadvantage with this approach is that if the needle is advanced toward the opposite side of the lesion, medication may be administered in the nonaffected side.[13]

INTERLAMINAR EPIDURAL STEROID INJECTIONS

Interlaminar epidural steroid injections have also been demonstrated to be effectively performed under ultrasound guidance. In the long-axis plane, a parasagittal oblique view is obtained to identify the interlaminar space.[15] The transducer is then rotated into the short-axis plane to identify the epidural space, spinal canal, and posterior aspect of the vertebral body (**Fig. 7**). Once the interlaminar space is visualized, a Tuohy needle is inserted and advanced until loss of resistance (LOR) is felt. Evansa and colleagues[15] compared the accuracy and functional improvement in the use of ultrasound-guided interlaminar epidural steroid injection with fluoroscopic control. Once LOR was reached with negative aspiration, contrast was injected and spread of injectate was confirmed under fluoroscopy. After confirmation of contrast spread, a mixture of 4 mL of 1% lidocaine and 80 mg of methylprednisolone was injected. This study demonstrated greater success rate in achieving epidural puncture during the first needle insertion in the ultrasound group. Both groups experienced similar improvements in pain and functional status.[15] Although further, larger-scale research needs to be performed to validate the accuracy of this approach, positive outcomes suggest that ultrasound-guided interlaminar injections may be considered an option for the interventionalist.

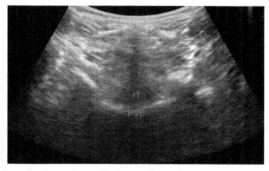

Fig. 7. Transverse interlaminar view. ISL, interspinous ligament; IT, intrathecal space; PVB, posterior vertebral body. (*Courtesy of* Allen S. Chen, MD, MPH, New York, NY.)

LUMBAR TRANSFORAMINAL INJECTIONS

The use of ultrasound for performing transforaminal injections is still developing, and recent studies demonstrate that it may be a feasible alternative to other image-guided modalities. However, numerous barriers remain. When performing lumbar transforaminal injections under ultrasound, a clear demonstration of lumbar anatomy and its associated landmarks is pivotal for ensuring accuracy and safety. There are several important structures to recognize when conducting ultrasound-guided transforaminal injections–the spinous process, vertebral lamina, facets, transverse process, and vertebral isthmus.[16] Another key landmark to identify is the intertransverse ligament, which extends from the upper border of one transverse process to the lower border of the according transverse process above.[16] This ligament has been described in several studies as a target structure for enhancing the feasibility and accuracy of ultrasound-guided transforaminal injections. The posterior foraminal approach and oblique approach are 2 notable techniques demonstrated in literature.[16,17] Given various approaches, sonoanatomic landmarks, and potential risks associated with transforaminal injections, it is recommended that ultrasound-guided transforaminal injections are performed only by seasoned practitioners with extensive ultrasound injection experience.

SACROILIAC JOINT INJECTIONS

SI joint-mediated pain is a common source of low back pain with reported prevalence rates of 10% to 30%.[18–20] The SI joint is a large diarthrodial joint with a fibrous posterosuperior component and a synovial anteroinferior component. Therefore, the more caudal aspect of the SI joint is representative of true synovium and is a frequently targeted site for SI joint injections.[21,22] Because of its complexity, image guidance is often necessary to reliably inject the SI joint. In a study by Rosenberg and colleagues,[23] it was found that clinically guided SI joint injections without any image localization have an intra-articular injection success rate of only 22%. Further details regarding the SI joint and associated interventional procedures are discussed in David A Soto Quijano's article, "Sacroiliac Joint Interventions," in this issue.

Technique

The technique and feasibility of ultrasound-guided SI joint injections were first described by Pekkafahli and colleagues.[21] First, the patient is placed in prone positioning with the probe placed in the short-axis plane in the sacral region. During the initial scan, several important bony landmarks are identified for orientation: the bony contours of the PSIS laterally and the spinous process of the fifth lumbar vertebrae medially.[22,24] Although moving the probe caudad, the next structures to visualize are the dorsal surface of the sacrum, medial and lateral sacral crest, gluteal surface of the ilium, and the first and second posterior sacral foramen. One method of identifying the SI joint starts by first placing the probe over the spinous process of the fifth lumbar vertebrae and scanning caudally over the medial sacral crest until the second posterior foramen is visible.[22] At this position, the SI joint is then observed as a hypoechoic cleft between the 2 echogenic lines of the sacrum and iliac bone[21] (**Fig. 8**). The cleft is scanned further caudally until it reaches the end of the iliac bone. Once these landmarks are identified, the probe should be over the distal third of the SI joint, where the needle is inserted.

In order to avoid intravascular injection, color Doppler ultrasound can be used for identifying the presence of vascular structures in or around the SI joint.[19,22] Once the target site is delineated, a spinal needle enters approximately 1 cm above the lower third of the hypoechoic cleft and approximately 2 cm medial to the line of the

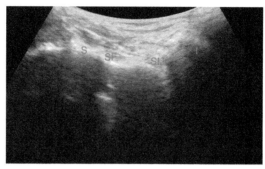

Fig. 8. Right SI joint. I, ilium; S, sacrum; SF, sacral foramen; SIJ, sacroiliac joint. (*Courtesy of* Allen S. Chen, MD, MPH, New York, NY.)

of the SI joint.[21] This needle entry angle from medial to lateral runs parallel with the joint's axis, as the cleft generally runs in a medial to lateral orientation proximally and runs more vertically distally.[24] The needle is further advanced until it reaches the posterior ligament. After correct needle positioning, a mixture of anesthetic and corticosteroid is then injected.

In Pekkafahli and colleagues'[21] study, 60 SI joints were injected in 34 patients with sacroiliitis, with a reported 76.7% success rate of intra-articular injections. Interestingly, the intra-articular rate was 60% in the first 30 injections, and 93.5% in the last 30 injections, further suggesting that accuracy may be directly related to experience and frequency of exposure.[21]

Another study by Klauser and colleagues[24] compared the success of performing ultrasound-guided SI joint injections using 2 different approaches: the upper level represented by the first sacral foramen and the lower level represented by the second sacral foramen. Klauser showed that the target was successfully reached at the upper level in 70% of injections and at the lower level in 90% of the injections using CT confirmation.[24] In a smaller subset of patients, the caudal cleft was not clearly defined, and thus, the upper approach was used for better visualization. The results from this study demonstrated an overall higher success rate with the lower level approach.[24] Other advantages of using the lower level of the SI joint as the target site include its more superficial location and vertical orientation, allowing for an easier needle trajectory.[24] In cases in which the lower level is not clearly visualized due to bony obstruction, the upper level of the joint can be considered a potential target.

SUMMARY

As ultrasonography grows in popularity, it has proven to be a useful and promising tool for the spine interventionalist. It should be considered part of a multimodal approach to patient care. Providers should weigh advantages and disadvantages when compared with other image-guided procedures, such as fluoroscopy and CT. Further studies evaluating safety, efficacy, and comparisons of ultrasound to other image-guided procedures are needed.

REFERENCES

1. Marhofer P, Chan VW. Ultrasound-guided regional anesthesia: current concepts and future trends. Anesth Analg 2007;104(5):1265–9.

2. Sites BD, Spence BC, Gallagher J, et al. Regional anesthesia meets ultrasound: a specialty in transition. Acta Anaesthesiol Scand 2008;52(4):456–66.
3. Provenzano DA, Narouze S. Sonographically guided lumbar spine procedures. J Ultrasound Med 2013;32(7):1109–16.
4. Wu T, Zhao WH, Dong Y, et al. Effectiveness of ultrasound-guided versus fluoroscopy or computed tomography scanning guidance in lumbar facet joint injections in adults with facet joint syndrome: a meta-analysis of controlled trials. Arch Phys Med Rehabil 2016;97(9):1558–63.
5. Yang G, Liu J, Ma L, et al. Ultrasound-guided versus fluoroscopy-controlled lumbar transforaminal epidural injections: a prospective randomized clinical trial. Clin J Pain 2016;32(2):103–8.
6. Greher M, Scharbert G, Kamolz LP, et al. Ultrasound-guided lumbar facet nerve block: a sonoanatomic study of a new methodologic approach. Anesthesiology 2004;100(5):1242–8.
7. Greher M, Kirchmair L, Enna B, et al. Ultrasound-guided lumbar facet nerve block: accuracy of a new technique confirmed by computed tomography. Anesthesiology 2004;101(5):1195–200.
8. Shim JK, Moon JC, Yoon KB, et al. Ultrasound-guided lumbar medial-branch block: a clinical study with fluoroscopy control. Reg Anesth Pain Med 2006; 31(5):451–4.
9. Greher M, Moriggl B, Peng PW, et al. Ultrasound-guided approach for L5 dorsal ramus block and fluoroscopic evaluation in unpreselected cadavers. Reg Anesth Pain Med 2015;40(6):713–7.
10. Galiano K, Obwegeser AA, Bodner G, et al. Ultrasound guidance for facet joint injections in the lumbar spine: a computed tomography-controlled feasibility study. Anesth Analg 2005;101(2):579–83.
11. Gofeld M, Bristow SJ, Chiu S. Ultrasound-guided injection of lumbar zygapophyseal joints: an anatomic study with fluoroscopy validation. Reg Anesth Pain Med 2012;37(2):228–31.
12. Galiano K, Obwegeser AA, Walch C, et al. Ultrasound-guided versus computed tomography-controlled facet joint injections in the lumbar spine: a prospective randomized clinical trial. Reg Anesth Pain Med 2007;32(4):317–22.
13. Park Y, Lee JH, Park KD, et al. Ultrasound-guided vs. fluoroscopy-guided caudal epidural steroid injection for the treatment of unilateral lower lumbar radicular pain: a prospective, randomized, single-blind clinical study. Am J Phys Med Rehabil 2013;92(7):575–86.
14. Park KD, Kim TK, Lee WY, et al. Ultrasound-guided versus fluoroscopy-guided caudal epidural steroid injection for the treatment of unilateral lower lumbar radicular pain: case-controlled, retrospective, comparative study. Medicine (Baltimore) 2015;94(50):e2261.
15. Evansa I, Logina I, Vanags I, et al. Ultrasound versus fluoroscopic-guided epidural steroid injections in patients with degenerative spinal diseases: a randomised study. Eur J Anaesthesiol 2015;32(4):262–8.
16. Loizides A, Peer S, Plaikner M, et al. Ultrasound-guided injections in the lumbar spine. Med Ultrason 2011;13(1):54–8 [Erratum appears in Med Ultrason 2011;13(2):178].
17. Galiano K, Obwegeser AA, Bodner G, et al. Real-time sonographic imaging for periradicular injections in the lumbar spine: a sonographic anatomic study of a new technique. J Ultrasound Med 2005;24(1):33–8.
18. Perry JM, Colberg RE, Dault SL, et al. A cadaveric study assessing the accuracy of ultrasound-guided sacroiliac joint injections. PM R 2016;8(12):1168–72.

19. Soneji N, Bhatia A, Seib R, et al. Comparison of fluoroscopy and ultrasound guid-ance for sacroiliac joint injection in patients with chronic low back pain. Pain Pract 2016;16(5):537–44.

20. Hurdle MF. Ultrasound-guided spinal procedures for pain: a review. Phys Med Rehabil Clin N Am 2016;27(3):673–86.

21. Pekkafahli MZ, Kiralp MZ, Başekim CC, et al. Sacroiliac joint injections performed with sonographic guidance. J Ultrasound Med 2003;22(6):553–9.

22. Jee H, Lee JH, Park KD, et al. Ultrasound-guided versus fluoroscopy-guided sacroiliac joint intra-articular injections in the noninflammatory sacroiliac joint dysfunction: a prospective, randomized, single-blinded study. Arch Phys Med Rehabil 2014;95(2):330–7.

23. Rosenberg JM, Quint TJ, de Rosayro AM. Computerized tomographic localiza-tion of clinically-guided sacroiliac joint injections. Clin J Pain 2000;16(1):18–21.

24. Klauser A, De Zordo T, Feuchtner G, et al. Feasibility of ultrasound-guided sacro-iliac joint injection considering sonoanatomic landmarks at two different levels in cadavers and patients. Arthritis Rheum 2008;59(11):1618–24.

Peripheral Nerve Radiofrequency Neurotomy: Hip and Knee Joints

Liza Hernández-González, MD*, Carlos E. Calvo, MD,
David Atkins-González, MD

KEYWORDS

- Genicular • Radiofrequency • Neurotomy • Hip pain • Knee pain • Osteoarthritis

KEY POINTS

- Osteoarthritis in the hip and knee joints is associated with joint pain, stiffness, weakness, and limited ambulation, which leads to significant psychosocial and physical disability.
- Intra-articular causes of hip pain can be successfully treated with radiofrequency neurotomy of the articular branches of the femoral and obturator nerves with minimal complications.
- Radiofrequency neurotomy of the knee can improve pain and function in patients with knee osteoarthritis.

INTRODUCTION

Osteoarthritis (OA) is the most common joint disorder in the general population.[1–3] Multiple modifiable and nonmodifiable risk factors play a role in its development and progression, particularly in the weight-bearing joints. These factors include old age, female gender, obesity, previous knee injury, repetitive overload, muscle weakness, joint laxity, effusion, and synovitis, among others.[3–6] It is associated with joint pain, stiffness, quadriceps weakness, impaired ambulation, and sleep disturbances, leading to significant psychosocial and physical disability.[7–12]

Nonsurgical treatment alternatives recommended for the management of hip and knee OA include education, exercise, physical therapy, topical agents, acetaminophen, nonsteroidal anti-inflammatory drugs, intra-articular injection with corticosteroids, hyaluronic acid, regenerative medicine and acupuncture, among others.[13–15] Some patients with severe incapacitating disease, however, may not respond to these alternatives due to either low efficacy, increased adverse effects, or severity of

Disclosure Statement: The authors have nothing to disclose.
Rehabilitation Medicine Service, VA Caribbean Healthcare System, 10 Casia Street, San Juan, PR 00921, USA
* Corresponding author.
E-mail address: lhernandezpmr@gmail.com

Phys Med Rehabil Clin N Am 29 (2018) 61–71
https://doi.org/10.1016/j.pmr.2017.08.006
1047-9651/18/Published by Elsevier Inc.
pmr.theclinics.com

disease. Even though surgical management is an alternative, some patients may not be candidates due to increased risk of surgery secondary to their comorbid diseases or simply may not wish to undergo surgery.

Radiofrequency (RF) neurotomy has been described as a treatment alternative for chronic peripheral joint pain.[16–18] RF has been extensively studied for the treatment of chronic pain conditions, such as spinal facet joint-mediated pain, sacroiliac joint pain, radiculopathy, and trigeminal neuralgia, among others.[19,20] It may be performed by different lesioning methods, including conventional RF (CRF), pulsed RF (PRF), and cooled RF, described later. RF neurotomy might be considered a successful alternative treatment with few complications for patients with chronic knee or hip OA who have a poor response to conservative management or are not candidates for surgery.

HIP JOIŃT PAIN
Anatomy

The hip joint is a true synovial, ball-and-socket joint between the acetabulum and the head of the femur. Its static stability originates mostly from its bony configuration and soft tissue attachments, especially on the anterior aspect of the joint capsule. It has a multiplanar range of motion facilitated by the activation of adjacent muscles.

The sensory innervation of the hip joint capsule originates primarily from the lumbosacral plexus and peripheral nerve branches, including the femoral, obturator, sciatic, and superior gluteal nerves. Based on anatomic and radiologic studies, it has a complex innervation divided into anterior and posterior aspects.[21–23] The anterior hip joint is predominantly innervated by articular branches of the obturator nerve anteromedially and the femoral nerve anterolaterally. Significant anatomic variations have been found on the obturator nerve, including an accessory nerve, variable number of articular branches, and width of distribution.[21–23] On its posterior aspect, it has major contributions from the sciatic nerve and nerve to quadratus femoris posteromedially, and superior gluteal nerve posterolaterally[21] (**Fig. 1**).

Microscopically, studies have found that the highest areas of free sensory nerve endings are located at the anterior and superior aspects of the hip joint capsule, especially at its anteromedial aspect.[22] Other studies evaluating the innervation of the human acetabular labrum have found more abundant free nerve endings on its superficial anterior-superior and posterior-superior zones.[24] Fewer studies have evaluated the presence of sensory nerve endings and mechanoreceptors on the posterior hip joint and have described a minimal amount of sensory nerve fibers in this area.[25,26] These findings may explain the variable pain referral patterns of patients with hip pathology predominantly reported to the groin and anteromedial thigh but also buttock, knee, and distal lower leg.[27,28]

Indications

Hip pain is a common complaint in the general population and causes may vary with age. Potential pain generators include intra-articular and extra-articular structures, such as the joint capsule ligaments, labrum, synovium, bone, bursae, tendons, and nerves. A specific pathoanatomic diagnosis of hip pain is sometimes difficult to establish due to multiple pain generators and variable hip pain referral patterns (groin, trochanteric, thigh, and buttock pain) as well as referred pain from other anatomic locations (low back, pelvic viscera, and peripheral nerves).[27,28] For these reasons, some studies have suggested the use of intra-articular injections[29–33] and/or diagnostic blocks of the articular branches of the obturator and femoral nerves to differentiate intra-articular causes of hip pain from extra-articular causes, including hip pain of

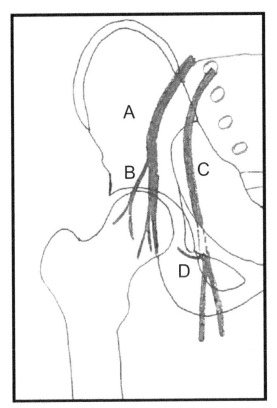

Fig. 1. Sensory innervation of the hip. (A) Femoral nerve, (B) articular nerve branch of the femoral nerve, (C) obturator nerve, and (D) articular nerve branch of the obturator nerve.

spinal origin.[34–37] The analgesic efficacy for corticosteroid injections or nerve blocks, however, has a short-term to intermediate-term duration of up to 12 weeks.[33,36]

RF neurotomy has been reported as a useful treatment alternative for patients with persistent hip pain who fail conservative measures or have short-term response to therapeutic injections. It may also be used to provide longer term analgesia in patients with significant comorbid disease who are not surgical candidates or those who want to delay surgery or are unwilling to perform surgery. Common diagnostic uses reported in the literature are OA, bone malignancy, avascular necrosis of the hip, fractures, and persistent postarthroplasty pain, among others.[35,38–46] Outcomes in several prospective studies have shown improved pain up to 11 months, decreased pain medication consumption, and improved patient function.[42,44] Most studies published, however, include case reports and retrospective studies with only 2 prospective studies. There is also a lack of studies evaluating RF lesioning on patients with pain in buttock distribution originated from posterior hip nerves.

Technique

RF denervation for chronic persistent hip pain is commonly performed by lesioning the articular branches of the obturator and femoral nerves. Traditionally, fluoroscopy guidance has been used to guide needle placement into the anatomic landmarks described for these nerves. The patient is placed in a supine position and an AP fluoroscopic view is obtained of the hip joint to be treated. The AP and oblique approaches have been described for lesioning the articular branches of the obturator nerve, the former the most commonly used. The anterolateral approach has been described to perform neurotomy of the articular branches of the femoral nerve.

The AP approach accesses the articular branches of the obturator nerve medial to the femoral artery and under the inguinal ligament.[38,39] The femoral artery is palpated and the skin is marked. The target zone is located at the inferior junction of ischium and pubis (teardrop shape on anteroposterior [AP] view). Then, an RF cannula is inserted perpendicularly under AP fluoroscopic guidance until bony contact is made. For lesioning the articular branches of the femoral nerve, the skin is accessed by the anterolateral approach 2 cm to 3 cm lateral to the femoral artery. The target zone is located at the superomedial aspect of the acetabulum below the anterior inferior iliac spine and near the anterolateral margin of the hip joint. The RF cannula is inserted on AP fluoroscopic guidance and directed until bony contact is made[39] (**Fig. 2**).

Some studies have argued, however, that the effectiveness of an AP approach for nerve lesioning may be low because the RF cannula contacts the target nerve in a perpendicular fashion (single lesion), which does not circumvent the challenges for potential anatomic nerve variations. As per clinical studies, a parallel orientation of the RF cannula to the target nerve is desired to increase the potential for multiple lesions on the target nerve to account for previously described anatomic variations, especially the obturator nerve.[22,47] In addition, cadaveric studies have estimated puncture of femoral vein and artery in 55% of the cases (N = 11/20), which has also been reported as a complication in several studies using this approach.[22,42,44,45]

More recently, the oblique approach uses the same target zones for the articular branches of the obturator nerve. It was developed to provide better electrode alignment with the target nerve (parallel orientation) and produce multiple lesions as well as minimize injury to neurovascular structures.[22] To access the articular branches of the obturator nerve, a 22-g spinal needle is inserted as a guide medial to the femoral artery under AP fluoroscopic guidance to the teardrop shape until bony contact is made. Then, the C-arm is rotated 60° to 70° ipsilateral and 20° cephalad to optimize parallel orientation of the RF cannula to the nerve and direct the needle posterior or deep to the neurovascular structures. After local anesthesia of the skin, the RF cannula is inserted in a tunnel view toward the tip of the guide spinal needle until bone contact

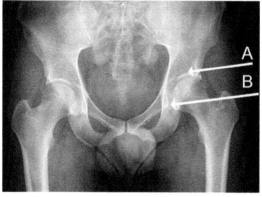

Fig. 2. AP view, hip radiographs. (A) Lesion site of the articular branch of the femoral nerve at the superomedial aspect of the acetabulum below the anterior inferior iliac spine and near the anterolateral margin of the hip. (B) Lesion site of the articular branch of the obturator nerve at the inferior junction of ischium and pubis (*teardrop shape*).

is made. At this point, some studies have suggested the use of combined fluoroscopy and ultrasound guidance to avoid damage of the neurovascular structures, especially for patients with difficult anatomy or large body habitus.[48,49] Once the target has been achieved, an AP view is then used to verify that the RF cannula remains lateral to the guide spinal needle. After placement of the RF electrode, sensory stimulation at 50 Hz is performed. Expected paresthesia should be elicited in the groin and hip region for the obturator nerve, and in the hip and lateral thigh for the femoral nerve. Threshold sensory stimulation for adequate electrode placement should be 50 Hz at less than 0.6 V. For safety precautions, motor stimulation may be performed at 2.0 Hz for up to 0.9 V while observing for absence of muscle activation in the lower extremity. After the expected responses are obtained, 1.5 mL to 2 mL of lidocaine 1% is injected per each cannula prior to nerve lesioning with CRF, PRF, or cooled RF.

The sensorimotor testing for optimal needle position is performed and, if confirmed, the guide needle is removed. Multiple site lesions maybe be performed in more caudal positions to produce additional lesions after proper sensorimotor testing at each site to avoid lesioning of the obturator nerve trunk.[22,50]

The denervation protocol has been described with CRF, PRF, and cooled RF methods. Conventional methods reported are variable in temperature (75°C–90°C), time of lesioning (90–180 seconds), and number of lesions per anatomic location (1–2 consecutive neurotomy lesions). PRF neurotomy has been used and justified due to the possible risks of neuritis and neuroma formation reported with CRF neurotomy.[41,44] Compared with CRF, these have been performed with lower temperatures (42°C), different lesioning times (120–180 seconds), and high-frequency alternating current. Only 1 case report was found using cooled RF of the articular branch of the femoral nerve in patients with chronic postarthroplasty hip pain, with significant pain relief and improved function up to 24 months.[46] Despite reports of possible complications with CRF, all methods used have shown short to long term analgesia (3–24 months) and improved function with minimal complications.

Complications

RF denervation of the articular branches of the femoral and obturator nerves seems a safe procedure with minimal complications, including transient hematoma formation due to blood vessel puncture and numbness in lateral thigh with RF lesioning using the anterior approach.[40,42,44,45]

KNEE JOINT PAIN
Anatomy

The knee joint is one of the largest and most complex in the body. It is formed by the femur, tibia, and patella along with multiple other structures, including ligaments and menisci. Its range of motion is mostly in flexion and extension (180°) along with minimal internal and external rotation (10°).

Knee innervation involves articular branches from the distal portions of the femoral, sciatic and obturator nerves. Franco and colleagues[51] concluded that innervation of the knee capsule can be divided into anterior and posterior. The anterior knee is innervated by anterior genicular branches derived from the femoral and common peroneal nerves. The posterior knee is innervated by the sciatic nerve, mostly its tibial branch. On some occasions, there is a component from the posterior branch of the obturator nerve.

Multiple studies describe the course of the genicular branches along different aspects of the knee.[51,52] There are 6 commonly described nerves.

- The superolateral branch is derived from the common peroneal nerve and courses close to the lateral epicondyle and the shaft of the femur. It provides distribution to the anterior superolateral aspect of the capsule.
- The middle genicular branch is derived from the tibial and travels through the vastus intermedius down to the anterior aspect of the distal femur.
- The superomedial branch also comes from the tibial nerve and is found close to the junction of the medial epicondyle and the shaft of the femur. It provides innervation to the superomedial aspect of the capsule.
- The inferolateral branch derives from the common peroneal nerve and courses beneath the fibular head, where it provides innervation to the inferolateral anterior aspect of the capsule.
- The lateral reticular nerve derives from the common peroneal nerve at the lateral side of the joint and provides innervation to the lateral aspect of the capsule.
- The inferomedial branch is derived from the tibial nerve and travels close to the medial condyle of the tibia and its shaft.

Indications

Genicular nerve RF neurotomy was initially described by Choi and colleagues,[16] who published a small double-blind randomized controlled trial in patients with severe chronic OA knee joint pain. It showed positive outcomes in terms of pain and function up to 12 weeks without adverse events. Thereafter, a systematic review was published with similar longer-term outcomes at 6 months in patients with chronic knee OA pain.[53] Saphenous neuralgia has been described due to persistent knee flexion in patients who undergo total knee replacement. RF lesioning of the saphenous nerve has been used in patients with persistent medial knee pain after total knee arthroplasty.[54] A more recent case report on patients with chronic postarthroplasty pain showed the patient had improved outcomes up to 3 months.[55] More studies are needed to evaluate further indications, because, theoretically, genicular nerves innervate the whole anterior capsule of the knee joint.

Technique

Cadaveric studies have shown that despite anatomic variations on the proximal course of the nerves, the distal portions are usually found in the same location.[51] These findings facilitate proper identification and needle placement during RF neurotomy procedures with image guidance, such as fluoroscopy or ultrasound.

Fluoroscopy-guided procedure

Most studies describe lesioning of the superolateral, superomedial, and inferomedial nerves. The inferolateral branch is not performed because of its proximity to the peroneal nerve and possible nerve injury with motor nerve involvement. The patient is placed on the fluoroscopy table in a supine position with the knee flexed 15° and draped in a sterile fashion. True AP view is obtained through fluoroscopic guidance. Skin and soft tissue are then anesthetized with lidocaine 1%. Then, the RF cannulas are advanced percutaneously to the respective areas of the superomedial, superolateral, and inferomedial genicular nerves until contact is made with periosteum, as described previously. After placement of the RF electrode, sensory stimulation at 50 Hz is done. For adequate placement confirmation, threshold for sensory stimulation should be less than 0.6 V. Due to anatomic variations, motor stimulation may be performed at 2.0 V while observing for absence of muscle activation in the lower extremity. After the expected response is obtained with sensory and motor stimulation, 1.5 mL to 2 mL of lidocaine 1% is injected per each cannula prior to nerve lesioning with CRF, PRF, or cooled RF (**Fig. 3**).

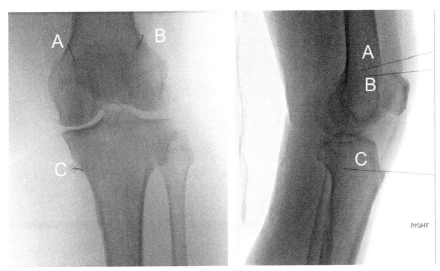

Fig. 3. AP (*left panel*) and lateral (*right panel*) views, knee radiographs. (A) Lesion site of the superomedial genicular nerve branch. (B) Lesion site of the superolateral genicular nerve branch. (C) Lesion site of the inferomedial genicular nerve branch.

Ultrasound-guided procedure

Ultrasound guidance may also be an alternative to fluoroscopy for genicular nerve diagnostic blocks before RF neurotomy. In cadaveric studies, ultrasound was found accurate for nerve location and, in theory, for better visualization of the neurovascular bundles compared to fluoroscopy.[52] The latter may vary, however, depending on equipment quality and operator-dependent skills due to the small size of the genicular neurovascular bundle. Yasar and colleagues[52] described an ultrasound-guided nerve block technique of the superomedial and inferomedial genicular nerves, which can be used as a guidance for neurotomy procedures. For the superomedial genicular nerve, the transducer is placed in a sagittal orientation over the femoral medial epicondyle and translated proximally to the adductor tubercle. The injection target is the bony cortex 1 cm anterior to the peak of the adductor tubercle using an in-plane approach (**Fig. 4**). To access the inferomedial genicular nerve, the transducer is placed in a sagittal

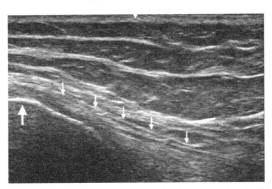

Fig. 4. Anatomic landmarks for superomedial genicular nerve block ([*large white arrow*] adductor tubercle of medial femoral condyle; [*small white arrows*] adductor magnus tendon). (*From* Yasar E, Kesikburun S, Kilik C, et al. Accuracy of ultrasound-guided genicular nerve block: a cadaveric study. Pain Physician 2015;18:E902; with permission.)

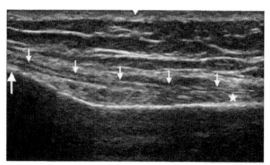

Fig. 5. Anatomic landmarks for inferomedial genicular nerve block ([*large white arrow*] tibial medial epicondyle; [*small white arrows*] medial collateral ligament; [*star*] insertion of medical collateral ligament). (*From* Yasar E, Kesikburun S, Kilik C, et al. Accuracy of ultrasound-guided genicular nerve block: a cadaveric study. Pain Physician 2015;18:E902; with permission.)

orientation over the tibial medial epicondyle to visualize the medial collateral ligament. The transducer is then translated distally to the tibial enthesis of the medial collateral ligament. Using an in-plane approach, the needle is directed to the midpoint between the peak of the tibial medial epicondyle and the fibers inserting on the tibial region of the medial collateral ligament (**Fig. 5**).

Complications

RF denervation of the genicular nerve branches for chronic knee OA pain seems a safe procedure with no adverse effects or complications reported. Kim and colleagues,[56] however, performed a literature review and anatomic study to establish its safety because genicular nerves travel near genicular arteries. These arteries provide blood supply to important structures, such as the distal femur, knee joint, meniscus, and patella. Even though reported vascular injury is uncommon and mostly reported after surgery, it may carry significant morbidities and must be considered when performing CRF neurotomy of the genicular nerves. These may include pseudoaneurysm formation, arteriovenous fistula, hemarthrosis, and osteonecrosis of the patella.

SUMMARY/RECOMMENDATIONS

Intra-articular hip and knee joint pathology is a common cause of pain and disability. Most conservative treatment options provide only short-term relief, especially for patients with severe intensity of pain. RF neurotomy of the hip and knee joints have shown to provide proper analgesia and improved function for short term and intermediate term with minimal to no complications. For these reasons, it may be a reasonable alternative for patients who have previously failed conservative treatment or are not surgical candidates. Nevertheless, more randomized controlled trials are necessary to evaluate its long-term efficacy and other possible indications.

REFERENCES

1. Helmick CG, Felson DT, Lawrence RC, et al. Estimates of the prevalence of arthritis and other rheumatic conditions in the United States. Part I. Arthritis Rheum 2008;58(1):15–25.

2. Lawrence RC, Felson DT, Helmick CG, et al. Estimates of the prevalence of arthritis and other rheumatic conditions in the United States. Part 2. Arthritis Rheum 2008;58:26–35.

3. Johnson VL, Hunter DJ. The epidemiology of osteoarthritis. Best Pract Res Clin Rheumatol 2014;28(1):5–15.

4. Barbour KE, Helmick CG, Boring M, et al. Vital signs: prevalence of doctor-diagnosed arthritis and arthritis-attributable activity limitation — United States, 2013–2015. Morb Mortal Wkly Rep 2017;66:246–53.

5. Barbour KE, Helmick CG, Boring M, et al. Obesity trends among adults with doctor-diagnosed arthritis— United States, 2009–2014. Arthritis Care Res 2017; 69(3):376–83.

6. Atukorala I, Kwoh CK, Guermazi A, et al. Synovitis in knee osteoarthritis: a precursor of disease? Ann Rheum Dis 2016;75(2):390–5.

7. McAlindon TE, Cooper C, Kirwan JR, et al. Determinants of disability in osteoarthritis of the knee. Ann Rheum Dis 1993;52(4):258–62.

8. McCurry SM, Von Korff M, Vitiello MV, et al. Frequency of comorbid insomnia, pain, and depression in older adults with osteoarthritis: predictors of enrollment in a randomized treatment trial. J Psychosom Res 2011;71:296–9.

9. Centers for Disease Control and Prevention. Prevalence of doctor-diagnosed arthritis and arthritis-attributable activity limitation: United States, 2010–2012. MMWR Morb Mortal Wkly Rep 2013;62:869–73.

10. Theis KA, Murphy L, Hootman JM, et al. Prevalence and correlates of arthritis-attributable work limitation in the US population among persons' ages 18–64: 2002 National Health Interview Survey data. Arthritis Rheum 2007;57:355–63.

11. Furner SE, Hootman JM, Helmick CG, et al. Health-related quality of life of US adults with arthritis: analysis of data from the behavioral risk factor surveillance system, 2003, 2005, and 2007. Arthritis Care Res 2011;63:788–99.

12. Centers for Disease Control and Prevention. Arthritis as a potential barrier to physical activity among adults with obesity. MMWR Morb Mortal Wkly Rep 2011;60:614–8.

13. Hochberg MC, Altman RD, April KT, et al. American College of Rheumatology 2012 Recommendations for the use of non-pharmacologic and pharmacologic therapies in osteoarthritis of the hand, hip, and knee. Arthritis Care Res 2012; 64(4):465–74.

14. Zhang W, Moskowitz RW, Nuki G, et al. OARSI recommendations for the management of hip and knee osteoarthritis, Part II: OARSI evidence-based, expert consensus guidelines. Osteoarthritis Cartilage 2008;16(2):137–62.

15. McAlindon TE, Bannuru RR, Sullivan MC, et al. OARSI guidelines for the non-surgical management of knee osteoarthritis. Osteoarthritis Cartilage 2014;22: 363–88.

16. Choi WJ, Hwang SJ, Song JG, et al. Radiofrequency treatment relieves chronic knee osteoarthritis pain: a double-blind randomized controlled trial. Pain 2011; 152:481–7.

17. Kesikburun S, Yasar E, Uran A, et al. Ultrasound-guided genicular nerve pulsed radiofrequency treatment for painful knee osteoarthritis: a preliminary report. Pain Physician 2016;19(5):E751–9.

18. Santana Pineda MM, Vanlinthout LE, Moreno Martín A, et al. Analgesic effect and functional improvement caused by radiofrequency treatment of genicular nerves in patients with advanced osteoarthritis of the knee until 1 year following treatment. Reg Anesth Pain Med 2017;42(1):62–8.

19. Byrd D, Mackey S. Pulsed radiofrequency for chronic pain. Curr Pain Headache Rep 2008;12(1):37–41.
20. Manchikanti L, Kaye AD, Boswell MV, et al. A systematic review and best evidence synthesis of the effectiveness of therapeutic facet joint interventions in managing chronic spinal pain. Pain Physician 2015;18(4):E535–82.
21. Birnbaum K, Prescher A, Hepler S, et al. The sensory innervation of the hip joint-An anatomical study. Surg Radiological Anat 1997;19:371–5.
22. Locher S, Burmeister H, Böhlen T, et al. Radiological anatomy of the obturator nerve and its articular branches: basis to develop a method for radiofrequency denervation for hip joint pain. Pain Med 2008;9(3):291–8.
23. Simons MJ, Amin NH, Cushner FD, et al. Characterization of the neural anatomy in the hip joint to optimize periarticular regional anesthesia in total hip arthroplasty. J Surg Orthop Adv 2015;24(4):221–4.
24. Alzaharani A, Bali K, Gudena R, et al. The innervation of the human acetabular labrum and hip joint: an anatomic study. BMC Musculoskelet Disord 2014; 15(41):1–8.
25. Dee R. Structure and function of the hip joint innervation. Ann R Coll Surg Engl 1952;45(6):357–74.
26. Gerdhart M, Johnson K, Atkinson R, et al. Characterization and classification of the neural anatomy in the human hip joint. Hip Int 2012;22(1):75–81.
27. Lesher JM, Dreyfuss P, Hager N, et al. Hip joint referral patterns: a descriptive study. Pain Med 2008;9(1):22–5.
28. Prather H, Hunt D, Fournie A, et al. Early intra-articular hip disease presenting with posterior pelvic and groin pain. PM R 2009;1:809–15.
29. Crawford RW, Gie GA, Ling RSM, et al. Diagnostic vale of intra-articular anesthetics in primary osteoarthritis of the hip. J Bone Joint Surg 1998;80-B:279–81.
30. Crawford RW, Gie GA, Ling RSM, et al. Intra-articular local anesthesia for pain after hip arthroplasty. J Bone Joint Surg 1997;79-B:796–800.
31. Odoom JE, Allen GM, Wilson DJ. Response to local anesthetic injections as a predictor of successful hip surgery. Clin Radiol 1999;54:430–3.
32. Kleiner JB, Thorne RP, Curd JG. The value of bupivacaine hip injection in the differentiation of coxarthrosis from lower extremity neuropathy. J Rheumatol 1991; 18:422–7.
33. Chandrasekaran S, Lodhia P, Suárez-Ahedo C, et al. Symposium: evidence for the use of intra-articular cortisone or hyaluronic acid injection in the hip. J Hip Preserv Surg 2015;3(1):5–15.
34. Hong Y, O'Grady T, Lopresti D, et al. Diagnostic obturator nerve block for inguinal and back pain: a recovered opinion. Pain 1996;67:507–9.
35. Fukui S, Nosaka S. Successful relief of hip joint pain by percutaneous radiofrequency nerve thermocoagulation in a patient with contraindications for hip arthroplasty. J Anesth 2001;15:173–5.
36. Yavuz F, Yasar E, Taskaynatan MA, et al. Nerve block of the articular branches of the obturator and femoral nerves for the treatment of hip joint pain. J Back Musculoskelet Rehabil 2013;26:79–83.
37. Cortiñas-Sáenz M, Salmerón-Vélez G, Holgado-Macho IA. Bloqueo intra-articular y de ramas sensoriales de los nervios obturador y femoral en cuadro de osteonecrosis y arthrosis de cabeza femoral. Rev Esp Cir Ortop Traumatol 2014; 58(5):319–24 [in Spanish].
38. Okada K. New approach to the pain of the hip joint. Pain Res 1993;8:125–35.

39. Kawaguchi M, Hashizume K, Iwata T, et al. Percutaneous radiofrequency lesioning of sensory branches of the obturator and femoral nerves for the treatment of hip joint pain. Reg Anesth Pain Med 2001;26:576–81.
40. Malik A, Simopolous T, Elkersh M, et al. Percutaneous radiofrequency lesioning of sensory branches of the obturator and femoral nerves for the treatment of non-operable hip pain. Pain Physician 2003;6:499–502.
41. Wu H, Groner J. Pulsed radiofrequency treatment of articular branches of the obturator and femoral nerves for management of hip joint pain. Pain Pract 2007;7(4):341–4.
42. Rivera F, Mariconda C, Annaratone G. Percutaneous radiofrequency denervation in patients with contraindications for total hip arthroplasty. Orthopedics 2012; 35(3):e302–5.
43. Kasliwali P, Iyer V, Kasliwali S. Percutaneous radiofrequency ablation for relief of pain in a patient of hip joint avascular necrosis. Indian J Pain 2014;28(2):121–3.
44. Chye C, Liang C, Lu K, et al. Pulse radiofrequency treatment of articular branches of femoral and obturator nerves for chronic hip pain. Clin Interv Aging 2015;10: 569–74.
45. Vanaclocha-Vanaclocha V, Sáiz-Sapena N, Herrera JM, et al. Percutaneous radiofrequency denervation in the treatment of hip pain secondary to osteoarthritis. EC Orthopaedics 2016;4(6):657–80.
46. Kim DJ, Shen S, Hanna GM. Ultrasound-guided radiofrequency lesioning of the articular branches of the femoral nerve for the treatment of chronic post-arthroplasty hip pain. Pain Physician 2017;20:E323–7.
47. Lord SM, Barnsley L, Wallis BJ, et al. Percutaneous radiofrequency neurotomy for chronic cervical zygapophyseal joint pain. N Engl J Med 1996;335:1721–6.
48. Chaiban G, Paradis T, Atallah J, et al. Use of ultrasound and fluoroscopy guidance in percutaneous radiofrequency lesioning of the sensory branches of the femoral and obturator nerves. Pain Pract 2014;4:343–5.
49. Stone J, Matchett G. Combined ultrasound and fluoroscopic guidance for radiofrequency ablation of the obturator nerve for intractable cancer-associated hip pain. Pain Physician 2014;17:E83–7.
50. Salmasi V, Chaiba G, Eissa H, et al. Application of cooled radiofrequency ablation in management of chronic joint pain. Tech Reg Anesth Pain Manag 2014;18: 137–44.
51. Franco C, Buvanendran A, Petersohn J, et al. Innervation of the anterior capsule of the human knee. Implications for radiofrequency ablation. Reg Anesth Pain Med 2015;40(15):363–8.
52. Yasar E, Kesikburun S, Kilik C, et al. Accuracy of ultrasound-guided genicular nerve block: a cadaveric study. Pain Physician 2015;18:E899–904.
53. Iannaccone F, Dixon S, Kaufman A. A review of long-term pain relief after genicular nerve radiofrequency ablation in chronic knee osteoarthritis. Pain Physician 2017;20(3):E437–44.
54. Clendenen S, Greengrass R, Whalen J, et al. Infrapatellar saphenous neuralgia after TKA can be improved with ultrasound-guided local treatments. Clin Orthop Relat Res 2015;473:119–25.
55. Protzman NM, Gyi J, Malhotra AD, et al. Examining the feasibility of radiofrequency treatment for chronic knee pain after total knee arthroplasty. PM R 2014;6:373–6.
56. Kim SY, Le PU, Kosharskyy B, et al. Is genicular nerve radiofrequency ablation safe? A literature review and anatomical study. Pain Physician 2016;19:E697–705.

Lumbar Epidural Steroid Injections

Carlos E. Rivera, MD

KEYWORDS

- Lumbar epidural steroid injections • Transforaminal • Interlaminar
- Epidural steroid injections techniques • Evidence

KEY POINTS

- Lumbar epidural steroid injections under fluoroscopic guidance are frequently used as part of the treatment of low back pain, especially with radicular component.
- Evidence shows these procedures are relatively safe and effective, especially for the short-term treatment of radicular pain.
- An adequate understanding of the relevant anatomy is important to be able to consistently deliver the injectate in the expected target and for safety considerations.
- Interlaminar and transforaminal approaches can be used to reach the epidural space. Each has different technical considerations that are discussed.

Low back pain is the leading cause of activity limitation and work absence throughout much of the world, imposing a high economic burden on individuals, families, communities, industry, and governments.[1] In the United States, back pain is the fifth most common reason individuals seek medical care and $30 to $50 billion in health care are spent on the treatment of this condition annually, with about 3% of emergency rooms visits.[2] Many of these subjects will develop chronic low back pain, adding to the individual and social cost. Globally, chronic low back pain has been estimated to have a prevalence of 4.2% in individuals aged between 24 and 39 years old and 19.6% in those aged between 20 and 59 years.[3] Point prevalence in different studies ranges from 12% to 33%, the 1-year prevalence ranged from 22% to 65%, and the lifetime prevalence ranges from 11% to 84%.[4]

Low back pain with radicular components is also very common and carries a worse prognosis in terms of pain, disability, chronicity, loss of productivity, quality of life, and use of health care resources, especially if the pain radiates to below the knee, indicating radiculopathy.[5,6] The annual prevalence in the general population, described as low back pain with leg pain traveling below the knee, varied from 9.9% to 25%, which means that it is presumably the most commonly occurring form of neuropathic pain.[7]

The author has nothing to disclose.
Campbell Clinic Orthopedics, 8000 Centerview Parkway, Suite 500, Memphis, TN 38138, USA
E-mail address: crivera@campbellclinic.com

Phys Med Rehabil Clin N Am 29 (2018) 73–92
https://doi.org/10.1016/j.pmr.2017.08.007
pmr.theclinics.com

Radicular pain is not always secondary to mechanical nerve compression as evidenced by patients with resolution of pain despite MRI findings of nerve compression, patients with no symptoms and abnormal studies, and patients without improvement in radicular pain after surgical decompression. The radicular nerve pain can be attributed to inflammatory and neurochemical mediators that act as principal modulators, if not precipitators, of the symptoms. These include phospholipase A2, neuropeptides such as substance P, vasoactive intestinal peptide, and calcitonin gene-related peptide that can be release from an injured nucleus. Increased local concentrations of these neuropeptides are thought to sensitize the free nerve endings, generating painful discharges, and producing back pain. It is also likely that these neuropeptides sensitize the adjacent nerve root and dorsal root ganglion, generating nerve root symptoms.[8] Treatment generally includes modifying activities, different exercise modalities, oral analgesics and neuropathic medications, physical therapy, manual manipulations, the use of epidural steroid injections, and, in certain, cases surgical interventions. Epidural injections can be performed via interlaminar, transforaminal, and caudal approaches injecting in isolation local anesthetic solutions, steroids, or a combination of both, and are commonly given to relieve pain and improve function and mobility, buying time for healing to occur. The exact mechanism of action of the drugs is not known and probably is multivariate, including an antiinflammatory effect, neural membrane stabilization effects, and the modulation of the peripheral nociceptor input.[9] In this article we will discuss the interlaminar and the transforaminal approaches.

ANATOMIC CONSIDERATIONS

- Understanding the anatomy of the lumbar spine is essential to perform accurate and safe lumbar epidural steroid injections. Special attention has to be given to the neurovascular structures in and around the epidural and foraminal areas.
- The epidural space is subdivided in a posterior and an anterior compartment.[9]
  - The anterior compartment is bordered anteriorly by the vertebral body, intervertebral disc, and the posterior longitudinal ligament, and posteriorly by the thecal sac; the posterior epidural space is bordered anteriorly by the thecal sac and posteriorly by the ligamentum flavum and the laminae. The diameter of the posterior space is about 5 to 6 mm from L2 to L5.
  - The contents of the epidural space include adipose tissue, loose areolar tissue, arteries, lymphatics, and an abundant venous plexus.
    - Fat cells are abundant in the dura that forms the sleeves around spinal nerve roots, but they are not embedded within the laminas that form the dura mater of the dural sac.[10]
    - Drugs stored in fat, inside dural sleeves, could have a greater impact on nerve roots than drugs stored in epidural fat, given that the concentration of fat is proportionally higher inside nerve root sleeves than in the epidural space, and that the distance between nerves and fat is shorter.[10]
- The intervertebral foramen
  - The intervertebral foramen is bordered anteriorly by the lower half of the upper of the 2 vertebral bodies, the intervertebral disc, and the upper half of the lower vertebral body, posteriorly by the facet joint, the lamina and ligamentum flavum, and superiorly and inferiorly by the pedicles of the adjacent vertebrae.
  - The exiting nerve root, lies high in the foramen (above the disc and below the pedicle) and is surrounded by the dural sleeve, which is composed of dura and arachnoid mater as far as the foramen.

○ Within the foramen, the dorsal and ventral nerve roots join into the spinal nerve
○ The spinal artery divides into several branches near the external opening of the foramen. A radicular branch joins the nerve root into the thecal sac. A spinal canal branch runs across the floor of the intervertebral foramen, along the sinuvertebral nerve that curves around the pedicle.
○ The rest of the foramen is fat.

EVIDENCE

- The clinical effectiveness and usefulness of epidural injections has been studied extensively, but differences in study designs, methodology, type of procedures, medications used, and diagnostic criteria make comparisons very difficult. Some early studies and reviews of non–fluoroscopically guided injections showed very poor success and no important benefits in comparing epidural steroid injections to intramuscular injections,[11] or to saline injections.[12] A systematic review of the effectiveness of non–image-guided lumbar interlaminar injections showed that it may have benefits for short-term pain relief (3–6 weeks).[13]
- The use of interlaminar and transforaminal epidural spinal injections has been corroborated by multiple studies and several reviews to provide reliable pain relief for patients with low back pain and radicular symptoms, but not axial back pain, with some long-term benefits lasting up to 12 months, and even surgery-sparing effects.[14–18]
- Studies seeking to identify patient characteristics to predict benefits have shown that patients with disc herniations or central stenosis, instead of other fixed lesions, single lesions, and higher baseline Oswestry Disability Index scores, have better outcomes.[19,20]
- Transforaminal versus interlaminar approaches
  ○ Another systematic review showed that both approaches could decrease pain and increase function with similar benefits at 6 months, but with some initial benefits (2 weeks) in pain relief for transforaminal.[21]
  ○ Good evidence that both can provide reliable pain relief for up to 6 months.[14]

INTERLAMINAR EPIDURAL STEROID INJECTIONS

- Interlaminar epidural injections deliver drugs to the epidural space for the treatment of low back pain, especially if radicular symptoms are present; interlaminar epidural access can also be use to place catheters or electrodes in the epidural space.[22] interlaminar epidural steroid injections are commonly used in general practice for the treatment of disc herniations and spinal stenosis with or without radicular pain, axial low back pain, and even for pain after fail surgical procedures.
  ○ The use of interlaminar epidural steroid injection for primarily axial pain, regardless of etiology, lacks effect[16] except possibly in short-term pain relief.[23]
  ○ For radicular pain secondary to disc herniations, the evidence is good with injections of steroids plus local anesthetics, and fair with local anesthetics only.[24]
  ○ The evidence is fair for radicular pain secondary to spinal stenosis.[24]
- Technique
  ○ Intravenous access is not necessary but is usually obtained in case of complications. No sedation is necessary and, in cases when it is used, like extreme anxiety, the patient should be able to be alert enough to carry conversation to avoid adverse events.

○ The patient is placed in a prone position with the face in a comfortable position to allow for clear communication. A pillow under the abdomen can help to flatten the lumbar lordosis and increase the opening of the interlaminar space.

○ The skin is cleansed in aseptic manner and covered in sterile drapes.

■ Two percent chlorhexidine in 70% alcohol is the preferred preparation for all spine procedures.[25]

○ Identify and optimize the segmental level you are targeting in an anteroposterior (AP) view by maximally opening the interlaminar space using a caudal or cephalad C-arm tilt (**Fig. 1**A).

○ Anesthetize the skin and soft tissue overlying the target point for painless insertion of the epidural needle (typically a Tuohy needle 18–22 gauge).

○ The target point should be the superior lamina of the lower vertebra in the segment (**Fig. 1**B).

■ Direct midline access should be avoided because the ligamenta flava can be separated by a space and you may miss the loss of resistance sensation. Direct insertion into the ligamentum flavum should also be avoided to be able to determine adequate depth of insertion and avoiding inserting needle to deep.

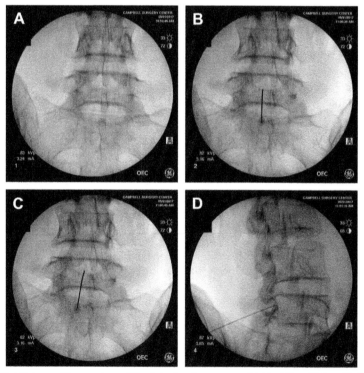

Fig. 1. (*A*) AP view with opening of the interlaminar space of L4 to L5 and L5 to S1. (*B*) Initial needle advancement targeting the superior border of the lamina from the lower vertebra in the segment. (*C*) Needle redirected to the ligamentum flavum. (*D*) Contralateral oblique view with needle just in the ligamentum flavum just at the interlaminar line. (*E*) Using loss of resistance to contrast dye in the contralateral oblique view. (*F*) Lateral view with contrast. (*G*) AP view with contrast. Optimally, the needle could be more lateral.

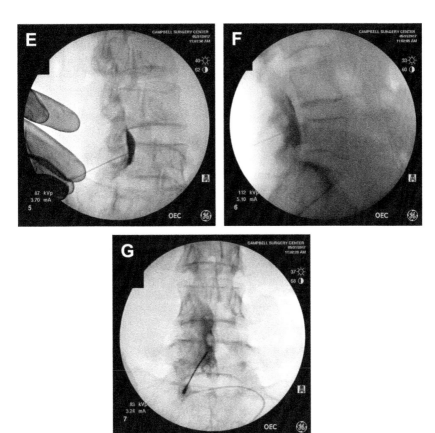

Fig. 1. (*continued*).

- Once the tip of the needle hits the superior lamina, it can be redirected to the ligamentum flavum (**Fig. 1**C). A loss of resistance syringe (with saline, air, or the contrast dye) is attached to the needle and the resistance of the ligament should be felt. If no resistance is felt, advance the needle millimeter by millimeter and test again.
- When resistance is perceived and while applying constant pressure on the syringe, the needle is slowly advanced until loss of resistance is obtained, and the needle is stopped.
- The C-arm should be turned into a lateral view to recheck depth of insertion. The needle should be in the posterior epidural space and seeing along the inferior articular process.
- A contralateral oblique view at around 45° can be used before the beginning loss of resistance (**Fig. 1**D). After redirecting the needle from the superior lamina to the ligamentum flavum the C-arm is turned to the contralateral oblique view that can provide better visualization of the needle tip and anatomic landmarks for safer advancement of the needle.[26] Loss of resistance can be attempted to access the epidural space in this view (**Fig. 1**E).
- Once the needle seems to be in the correct position, aspiration is attempted to check for blood or cerebrospinal fluid and, if negative, an extension tube

should be attached to the needle to avoid unnecessary movement. Then, contrast should be injected under live fluoroscopic visualization to check for vascular uptake or other abnormal uptake pattern. Contrast should be evident along the epidural space. The contrast should form a smooth but irregular pattern that seems to be somewhat lobulated, consistent with it permeating the epidural fat[27] (**Fig. 1F and G**).

- ○ Parasagittal access has shown to provide more effective pain relief than a midline approach at 6 months. Also, contrast spread to the ventral epidural space is higher.[28]
- ○ A modified interlaminar technique has been described that has shown better success than transforaminal injections accessing the ventral epidural space in cases of foraminal stenosis.[29]
- Medications
  - ○ Specific medication agents and doses vary among providers, and we lack studies comparing effectiveness.
  - ○ A combination of local anesthetics and corticosteroids is usually used and volumes typically range from 2 to 15 mL.
  - ○ Most common steroids used are triamcinolone, betamethasone, methylprednisolone, and dexamethasone.
  - ○ It is important to clarify that recently after an infection outbreak the US Food and Drug Administration release a safety alert stating that, "The effectiveness and safety of injection of corticosteroids into the epidural space of the spine have not been established, and [the US Food and Drug Administration] has not approved corticosteroids for this use."
- Pain provocation during injection
  - ○ Commonly during the injection of the agents the patient will experience pain in the back and/or the extremity.
  - ○ Sinofsky[30] showed that concordant pain provocation correlated with significantly higher pain reduction at 2 weeks, but this did not resulted in any significant difference in function or use of analgesics.
- Complications
  - ○ Infections, epidural hematomas, and allergic reactions are always considered, but very rare.
  - ○ Adrenal suppression from the use of steroids can last 2 to 3 weeks.[31]
  - ○ Headaches owing to dural puncture occur.
  - ○ Hypotension owing to sympathetic efferent blockade has been described in 2% to 3% of patients.

TRANSFORAMINAL EPIDURAL STEROID INJECTIONS
Indications

- Transforaminal injections are used for the treatment of radicular pain by injecting medication, usually corticosteroids, near the nerve roots. When using local anesthetic only, can also be used as a diagnostic test to determine if a specific spinal nerve is responsible for the patient's pain.
- The procedure goal is to apply the medication directly onto the affected spinal nerve in the intervertebral foramen that lodges the nerve, under radiographic control. The presumptions upon which the procedure is based are that using radiographic control would avoid missing the target nerve and that delivering the medication directly onto the affected nerve would maximize the prospective of having a therapeutic effect.[32]

Evidence

- MacVicar and colleagues[32] reviewed the literature and found that, in patients with radicular pain secondary to disc herniations, up to 70% of patients are at least 50% better at 1 to 2 months, and 40% of patients better at 12 months. Up to 30% experience complete pain relief. Patients with contained disc hernia-tions or low-grade compression have better results. Transforaminal epidural ste-roid injections are slightly less effective in chronic radicular pain. Transforaminal epidural steroid injections are better than caudal, interlaminar, and blind injections.[32]
- Another review of the literature concluded that there was strong evidence in the efficacy of the transforaminal approach in radicular pain.[33]
- Transforaminal epidural steroid injections help to reduce the burden of pain by increasing function and decreasing the need for other health care including surgery.[32]
- Roberts,[34] in another systematic review, concluded that there is fair evidence that transforaminal epidural steroid injections are superior to placebo for radic-ular symptoms, good evidence that it should be used as a surgery-sparing inter-vention, and that it is superior to interlaminar and caudal injections for radicular pain.

Subpedicular Transforaminal Injection Technique

- No sedation is necessary and in cases; when it is used, for example, for extreme anxiety, the patient should be able to be alert enough to carry conversation to avoid adverse events (**Figs. 2** and **3**).
- The patient is placed in a prone position with the face in a comfortable position to allow for clear communication.
- The skin is cleansed in aseptic manner and covered in sterile drapes
  - Two percent chlorhexidine in 70% alcohol as the preferred preparation for all spine procedures.[25]
- Identify and optimize the segmental level you are targeting in an AP view by squaring off the targeted segment lining up the superior endplate. This maneuver will usually require a cephalad tilt of the C-arm for the L4 to L5 and L5 to S1 seg-ments, and a caudal tilt for upper segments (see **Fig. 2**A).
- The target point is the posterior surface of the vertebral body near the midline (6 o'clock position or slightly lateral) aspect of the inferior border of the pedicle above the target nerve (see **Figs. 2**B and **3**A).
  - This is the so-called safe triangle area that is formed in the area between the lower margin of the pedicle. The nerve is unlikely to lie in the triangle unless it has been moved cephalad by foraminal stenosis.
  - To achieve an open look of the target point usually an ipsilateral oblique view is necessary. Following the Spinal Intervention Society guidelines, a minimal ob-lique rotation is used just enough to obtained a clear view of the target in which the margins of the superior articular process (SAP), the transverse process, and the lamina do not overlap.[35]
- Needle insertion will be on the area just inferior and lateral to the target point (**Fig. 3**B). Intermittent fluoroscopy is used to check that the needle is in the cor-rect path. If any deviation is observed, the needle is retracted slightly and the course is corrected. The needle can be steered by rotating the needle bevel and orienting it to the desired direction. Many practitioners also give a slight curve to the tip of the needle to have easier manipulation. The needle tip should always be in the safe triangle area.

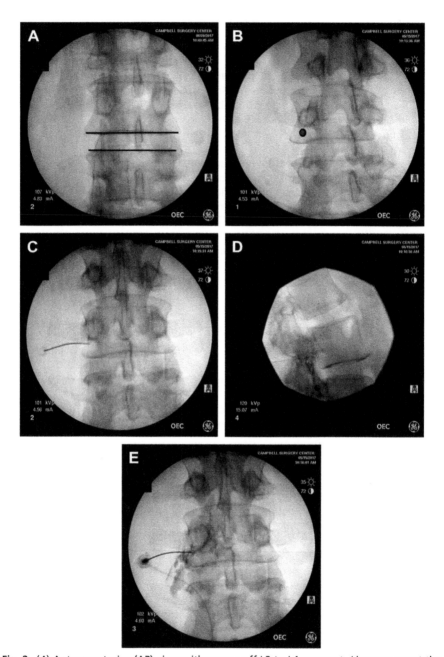

Fig. 2. (*A*) Anteroposterior (AP) view with square off L3 to L4 segment. *Lines* represent the lower and upper ring apophyses of the segment. (*B*) Target point (*blue oval*) in a slightly left oblique view. (*C*) AP view with needle tip lateral to the midline of the pedicle. (*D*) Lateral view with contrast. Needle in superoposterior aspect of the foramen just below the pedicle. (*E*) AP view with adequate contrast spread.

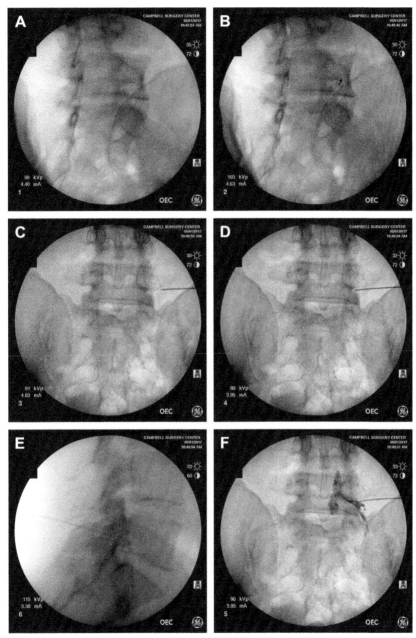

Fig. 3. (*A*) Oblique view to the right for initial needle insertion. (*B*) Needle insertion in oblique view targeting the bone for safety. (*C*) Anteroposterior (AP) view after touching bone. (*D*) Needle advancing in AP view just lateral to the midline of the pedicle. (*E*) Lateral view with contrast. Optimally, the needle could be more posterior in the foramen. (*F*) AP view with adequate contrast spread.

- Once the bone is contacted, turn the C-arm to an AP view to confirm that the needle tip is not medial to the midline of the pedicle (see **Figs. 2**C and **3**C and D). Then, a lateral view is obtained and the needle tip should be posterior to the vertebral body just below the pedicle (see **Figs. 2**D and **3**E). Staying in the posterior half of the foramen is recommended because most of the time vascular structures like the radicular artery and the intervertebral vein are found in the anterior part of the foramen just dorsal to the vertebral body.
- After the target point is reached, connect an extension tube to the syringe with contrast dye to avoid unnecessary movement and under live fluoroscopy inject slowly. Contrast flow should ideally outline the spinal nerve and then flow into the epidural space medial to the pedicle (see **Figs. 2**E and **3**F).
  - Even though is not a contraindication and trying to readjust the needle is an option, Spinal Intervention Society guidelines recommends to terminate the procedure if arterial or intrathecal flow is observed as a wise and safe option to avoid possible complications. If intravenous flow is observed, then readjusting the needle and retesting is advised.
  - Smuck and colleagues[36] found that the risk of simultaneous epidural and vascular injection is twice as likely to occur as vascular injection alone (9% vs 4%). Intermittent fluoroscopy can miss the transient appearance of the vascular component; therefore, live fluoroscopy is recommended when the contrast is injected.
- Finally, the medication agents are injected. The amount of agents to be injected vary with practitioners, but in general 4 mL of injectate reaches both the superior aspect of the superior intervertebral disc and the inferior aspect of the inferior intervertebral disc 93% of the time.[37] A comparative study showed that a volume of injectate of 8 mL was more effective than 3 mL for radicular pain, even when the dose of the steroid remained the same.[38]

Infraneural Transforaminal Injection Technique

- No sedation is necessary and, in cases when it is used, for example, for extreme anxiety, the patient should be able to be alert enough to carry conversation to avoid adverse events (**Figs. 4** and **5**)
- Patient positioning and skin preparation are the same as in the subpedicular approach.
- The goal is to place the tip of the needle just posterior to the disc in the inferior third of the foramen in what is known as Kambin's triangle (see **Fig. 4**A).
  - Kambin's triangle is defined as a right triangle over the dorsolateral disc. The hypotenuse is the exiting nerve root, the base (width) is the superior border of the caudal vertebra and the height is the traversing nerve root. This area can protect the needle tip from entering neural and vascular structures.[39,40]
  - In a study by Murthy and associates[41] looking at spinal angiograms, the radiculomedullary arteries were in the superior half of the foramen 97% of the time and never in the lower fifth. Also, the radiculomedullary arteries were in the left side 88% of the time.
- Using an AP projection, identify and optimize the segmental level being targeted in an AP by squaring off the targeted segment lining up the superior endplate. This maneuver usually requires a cephalad tilt of the C-arm for the L4 to L5 and L5 to S1 segments, and a caudal tilt for upper segments (see **Figs. 4**B and **5**A).
- Then, an ipsilateral oblique view is obtained so that the medial part of the SAP is seeing in the middle or slightly lateral to the middle of the disc (see **Figs. 4**C and **5**B).

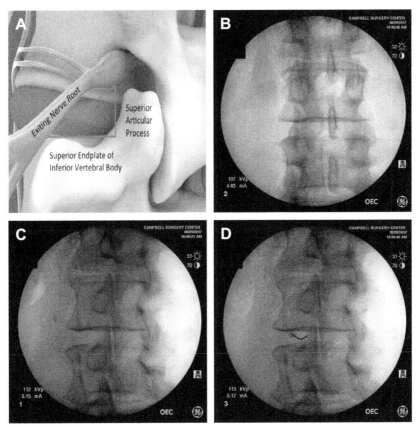

Fig. 4. (*A*) Kamin triangle. (*B*) Anteroposterior (AP) view with square off the L3 to L4 segment. (*C*) Left oblique view for initial needle insertion. (*D*) Initial needle advancement targeting the lower half of the superior articular process. (*E*) This is a lateral view after feeling bone contact in the ipsilateral oblique. (*F*) Needle advancing in the lateral view into the foramen. Needle in the inferoposterior half of the foramen. (*G*) Contrast injection in lateral view. (*H*) AP view with adequate contrast spread. ([*A*] *From* Abbasi H, Abbasi A. Oblique lateral lumbar interbody fusion (OLLIF): technical notes and early results of a single surgeon comparative study. Cureus 2015;7(10):3; with permission.)

- After inserting needle, it is directed to the lateral lower part of the SAP keeping the trajectory in the lower third of the foramen (for safety, it is recommended to hit the SAP; see **Figs. 4**D and **5**C). After this maneuver, turn the C-arm to a lateral position and slowly advance the needle into the posterior half of the foramen (see **Figs. 4**E and F, and **5**D and E).
- Initial contrast injection is done after connecting an extension tube to the needle (see **Figs. 4**G and **5**F). Owing to the location of the needle, inadvertent intradiscal injection can occur, especially in cases of foraminal disc herniations. If this is the case, slightly retract the needle and retest.
  - Inadvertent intradiscal injection can be expected in about 5% of cases and intrathecal spread in 3%.[42]
- Finally, turn the C-arm to an AP view and inject contrast dye again (see **Figs. 4**H and **5**G). The needle should not be medial to the 12 o'clock position of the inferior

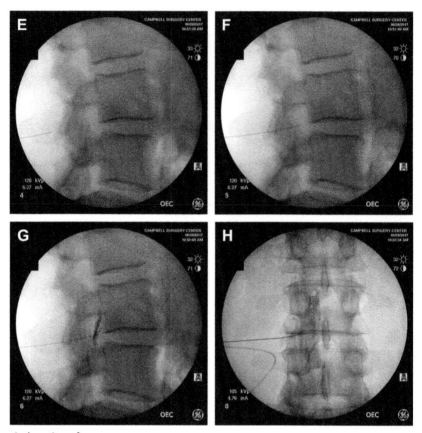

Fig. 4. (*continued*).

pedicle to avoid dural puncture; it should be in front of the zygopophysial joint shadow. Flow will be seen along the nerve and, very frequently, cephalad as the nerve transits inferiorly along the disc.[43]

○ Contrast should flow centrally across the disc interspace toward the midline, down around the pedicle below, and then at least along the proximal segmental nerve toward its foraminal entry. Contrast is more often than not seen flowing along the segmental nerve just above the needle as well. Contrast tends to flow into the central ventral and lateral epidural compartments. Contrast should at least initially be evident in the ventral epidural space under the lateral view and may outline an extrinsic mass effect or filling defect.[44]

○ Levi and Horn[42] found vascular infiltration in about 6.6% of cases in a retrospective review.

○ A volume of 3.0 mL of injectate reaches both the medial aspect of the inferior pedicle and the superior pedicle 94.6% of the time. Therefore, a 1-level instead of a 2-level injection for patients with a bleeding risk or for 2-level central pathology can be considered.[45]

○ Kim and coworkers,[46] injecting only 1 mL of contrast at the L4 level, found spread to the L4 nerve root in 90% of cases; at the L5 level, 60% reached the L5 nerve and 30% also the S1.

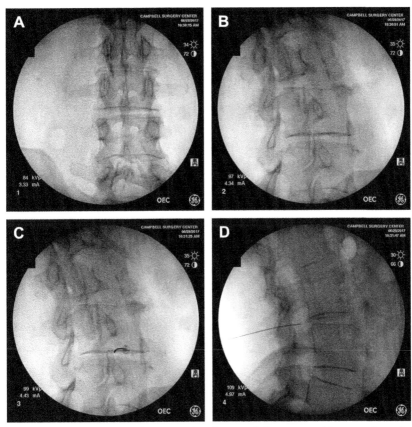

Fig. 5. (*A*) Anteroposterior (AP) view with suboptimal, but acceptable, squaring of end-plates at L3 to L4. (*B*) Right oblique view for initial needle insertion. (*C*) Initial needle advancement targeting the lower half of the superior articular process. (*D, E*) Advancing the needle in lateral view, keeping the needle in the inferior half of the foramen. (*F*) Lateral view during contrast administration. (*G*) AP view during contrast injection.

S1 SUBPEDICULAR TECHNIQUE

- The target point is on the caudal border of the S1 pedicle, just dorsal to the internal opening of the S1 anterior sacral foramen. It is reached by passing a needle through the posterior sacral foramen. The posterior foramen is not always easy to identify and can be confused with the anterior foramen that is usually larger are more obvious[47] (**Fig. 6**).
- Using a cephalad tilt, line up the sacral endplate. The posterior foramen is usually circular looking and its superior margin can overlap with the S1 pedicle.[47] Contrary to other transforaminal levels, a straight AP view can be used as the main needle trajectory view (see **Fig. 6**A).
- Insert the needle targeting to hit the sacrum to ensure adequate depth (see **Fig. 6**B). Once bone is contacted, the needle is readjusted superiorly and medially into the foramen (see **Fig. 6**C). The goal is to hit the caudal border of the anterior half of the S1 pedicle.[47] The spinal nerve is running in an inferolateral direction; therefore, keeping the needle tip medial is advised.

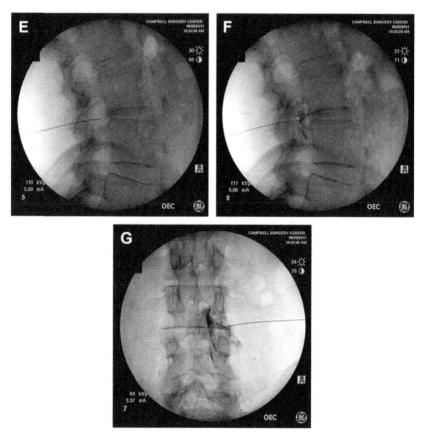

Fig. 5. (*continued*).

- After this, obtain a lateral view to make sure the needle is not to anterior (see **Fig. 6**D). In this view, the needle should never be ventral to the floor of the sacral canal. In optimal position, the tip of the needle should lie in contact superiorly with the middle of the caudal border of the S1 pedicle, at a depth within 5 mm of the floor of the sacral canal.[47]
- Connect the needle to the extension tube and slowly inject contrast dye under live fluoroscopy (see **Fig. 6**E). Contrast should flow outlining the spinal nerve, and nerve sheath, into the epidural space and continue cephalad. If vascular flow is seen, readjust the needle and retest or abort the procedure.
  - Two milliliters of contrast reach the media aspect of the S1 pedicle 100% of the time, 3 mL reached the superior aspect of the L5 to S1 segment more than 90% of the time.[48]
- Because it is not always easy to visualize the posterior sacral foramen a technique with a more oblique entry point can be used. Fish described it as the S1 "Scotty dog view." After lining up the sacral endplate, the C-arm is rotated ipsilateral oblique to view the L5 vertebral segment as a Scotty dog. When the L5 Scotty dog is visualized, the operator should view the S1 segment, and the dog's "neck" and forelimb can be visualized as the superomedial landmarks of the S1 foramen (even if the rest of the dog is not seen). The S1 SAP is the ear

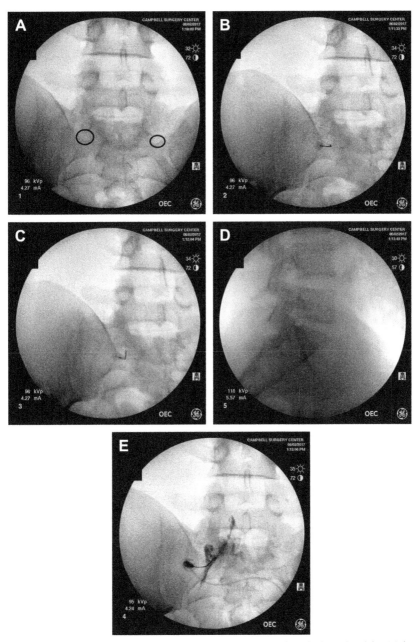

Fig. 6. (*A*) Anteroposterior (AP) view with S1 foramen inside the *black circles*. (*B*) Initial needle insertion targeting the sacrum near the inferior border of the foramen. (*C*) Needle redirected into the foramen. (*D*) Lateral view with contrast injection. (*E*) Injection of contrast in AP view. Observe the outlining of the nerve and the cephalad and medial spread.

of the S1 dog. The needle is aim to the hit bone for safety and then slipped into the foramen. The check depth of insertion AP and lateral views are obtained and as usual contrast dye is injected under direct fluoroscopic guidance[49] (**Fig. 7**).

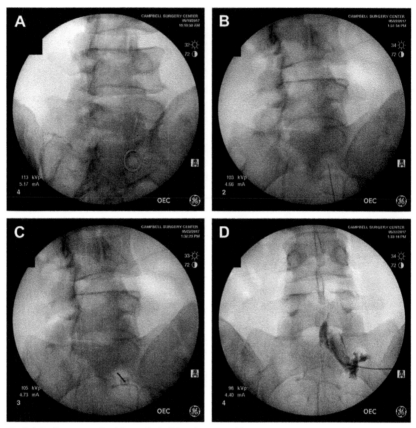

Fig. 7. (*A*) S1 foramen (inside *red circle*) using an oblique view. A more oblique position to obtain a better Scotty dog view of L5, as described in text, was impossible because it will have caused the iliac bone to obstruct with the needle trajectory. (*B*) Another oblique view to optimize view of the S1 foramen with needle tip marking the inferior wall. (*C*) Needle trajectory advancing into the foramen. (*D*) Contrast injection in anteroposterior view.

Other Considerations

- Postprocedure sensory changes in the distribution of the injected nerve are expected, as well as pain relief and even some temporary impairment of motor function.
  - Immediate postprocedure relief of pain does not strongly predict longer term effectiveness in pain relief or functional recovery. The response at 2 weeks is more strongly associated with the 2-month outcomes.[50]
- Subjects with a simultaneous epidural and vascular injection who returned for repeat injection had a statistically significant chance of a repeat simultaneous epidural and vascular injection when the injection was done at the same location.[36]
- The use of epidural steroid injections within 90 days of single level decompression should be carefully considered because some association has been found with the risk of postoperative infections and time interval of prior epidural steroid injections.[51]

Complications

- As part of the placement of the needle in the target zone, potential complications include the risk of infection and nerve damage. When following adequate technique, these events are extremely rare. Other complications are mainly owing to reactions to the injection agents.
- A multisite study of more than 16,000 procedures (mostly transforaminal) had no neurologic injuries, no hemorrhagic complications, and no infections. Vasovagal reactions were treated in 1.3% of transforaminal and 0.5% of interlaminar procedures. Transfers to the emergency departments were less than 0.1% and mainly related to allergic reactions and cardiovascular symptoms. Increased pain was described in about 2% of cases.[52]
- In another large sample, Plastaras[53] found a rate of minor adverse events both immediately and at 24 to 72 hours after the procedure, similar to that of other axial corticosteroid injections. Permanent adverse events were not found in their sample. Immediate and delayed adverse events occurred after 182 (9.2%) and 305 (20.0%) injections, respectively. Only 2 immediate adverse events occurred in more than 1% of procedures: vasovagal episode (4.2%) and intravascular flow that changed or interrupted the procedure (1.7%). Delayed adverse events that occurred in at least 1% of patients included pain exacerbation (5.0%), injection site soreness (3.9%), headache (3.9%), facial flushing and sweating (1.8%), and insomnia (1.6%).

USE OF ANTICOAGULANTS

- Holding the use of anticoagulant medications has been a standard practice when performing spinal procedures. Recently, this has been debated in terms of possible benefits, namely, decreasing the risk of epidural hematomas, of which there are no known reports causing neurologic damage after transforaminal epidural injections versus the risk of precipitating the thromboembolic events.
  - Antiplatelet medications have been shown not to be a significant hazard for the conduct of spinal pain procedures.[54,55]
  - The risk of morbidity by discontinuing anticoagulants seems to be greater than the adverse events possible from continuing it. Studies comparing patients who stop the anticoagulants versus those who continue have shown greater serious morbidity in those who stop the medications.[56]
  - Recently, this strategy has been debated in terms of possible benefits (decreasing the risk of epidural hematomas) versus the risk of precipitating thromboembolic events. Based on the risk–benefit ratio, Goodman and associates[57] created a guideline for spinal procedures based on previous recommendations from the Spinal Intervention Society and the American Society of Regional Anesthesia and Pain Medicine.

SUMMARY

Strong evidence exists of the benefit of lumbar epidural steroid injections in the treatment of lumbar radicular pain. We have discussed 3 different approaches—the interlaminar and 2 different transforaminal (subpedicular and infraneural). Guidelines from the Spinal Intervention Society were used as a basis for these technical recommendations. Even though these procedures are not a cure, its judicious use following evidence-based recommendations can provide benefit to patients suffering from this common problem, improve their function, and even have some surgery-sparing effects.

REFERENCES

1. Duthey B. Priority Medicines for Europe and the World "A public health approach to innovation" Update on 2004 background paper background paper 6.24 low back pain 15 March 2013.
2. Waterman BR. Low back pain in the United States: incidence and risk factors for presentation in the emergency setting. Spine J 2012;12(1):63–70.
3. Meucci RD, Fassa AG, Faria NMX. Prevalence of chronic low back pain: systematic review. Rev Saude Publica 2015;49:1.
4. Walker BF. The prevalence of low back pain: a systematic review of the literature from 1966 to 1998. J Spinal Disord 2000;13(3):205–17.
5. Spijker-Huiges A, Groenhof F, Winters JC, et al. Radiating low back pain in general practice: incidence, prevalence, diagnosis, and long-term clinical course of illness. Scand J Prim Health Care 2015;33(1):27–32.
6. Konstantinou K, Hider SL. The impact of low back-related leg pain on outcomes as compared with low back pain alone: a systematic review of the literature. Clin J Pain 2013;29(7):644–54.
7. Van Boxem K, Cheng J. Lumbosacral radicular pain. Pain Pract 2010;10(4): 339–58.
8. McLain RF, Kapural L. Epidural steroids for back and leg pain: mechanism of action and efficacy. Cleve Clin J Med 2004;71(12):961–70.
9. Sitzman BT. Epidural injections. In: Fenton D, editor. Image-guided spine intervention. Philadelphia: WB Saunders; 2003. p. 100–1.
10. Fyneface-Ogan S. Anatomy and Clinical Importance of the Epidural Space. In: Epidural Anesthesia - Current views and approaches. InTech 2012.
11. Wilson-MacDonald J. Epidural steroid injection for nerve root compression, a randomized, controlled trial. J Bone Joint Surg Br 2005;87:352–5.
12. Valat J, Giraudeau B, Rozenberg S, et al. Epidural corticosteroid injections for sciatica: a randomised, double blind, controlled clinical trial. Ann Rheum Dis 2003;62(7):639–43.
13. Vorobeychik Y. The effectiveness and risks of non–image-guided lumbar interlaminar epidural steroid injections: a systematic review with comprehensive analysis of the published data. Pain Med 2016;17:2185–202.
14. Landa J. Outcomes of interlaminar and transforminal spinal injections. Bull NYU Hosp Jt Dis 2012;70(1):6–10.
15. Okmen K. The efficacy of interlaminar epidural steroid administration in multilevel intervertebral disc disease with chronic low back pain: a randomized, blinded, prospective study. Spine J 2017;17:168–74.
16. Sharma AK. The effectiveness and risks of fluoroscopically guided lumbar interlaminar epidural steroid injections: a systematic review with comprehensive analysis of the published data. Pain Med 2017;18:239–51.
17. Bicket MC. Epidural injections in prevention of surgery for spinal pain: systematic review and meta-analysis of randomized controlled trials. Spine J 2015;15: 348–62.
18. Manchikanti L. Epidural injections for lumbar radiculopathy and spinal stenosis: a comparative systematic review and meta-analysis. Pain Physician 2016;19: E365–410.
19. Maus TP. Imaging determinants of clinical effectiveness of lumbar transforaminal epidural steroid injections. Pain Med 2016;17:2176–84.
20. Sivaganesan A. Predictors of the efficacy of epidural steroid injections for structural lumbar degenerative pathology. Spine J 2016;16:928–34.

21. Chang Chien GC. Transforaminal versus interlaminar approaches to epidural steroid injections: a systematic review of comparative studies for lumbosacral radicular pain. Pain Physician 2014;17:E509–24.

22. Bogduk N. Lumbar transforaminal access. In: Bogduk N, editor. Practice guidelines for spinal diagnostic and treatment procedures. San Francisco (CA): International Spine Intervention Society; 2013. p. 539.

23. DePalma MJ. Evidence-informed management of chronic low back pain with epidural steroid injections. Spine J 2008;8:45–55.

24. Benyamin RM, Manchikanti L, Parr AT, et al. The effectiveness of lumbar interlaminar epidural injections in managing chronic low back and lower extremity pain. Pain Physician 2012;15(4):E363–404.

25. Darouiche RO, Wall MJ, Itani KM, et al. Chlorhexidine-alcohol versus Povidone-iodine for surgical-site antisepsis. N Engl J Med 2010;362:18–26.

26. Gill JS, Nagda JV. Contralateral oblique view is superior to the lateral view for lumbar epidural access. Pain Med 2016;17(5):839–50.

27. Bogduk N. Lumbar transforaminal access. In: Bogduk N, editor. Practice guidelines for spinal diagnostic and treatment procedures. San Francisco (CA): International Spine Intervention Society; 2013. p. 548.

28. Ghai B, Vadaje KS. Lateral parasagittal versus midline interlaminar lumbar epidural steroid injection for management of low back pain with lumbosacral radicular pain: a double-blind, randomized study. Anesth Analg 2013;117(1): 219–27. Spine Journal, Volume 13(11): 1710.

29. Kim ED. Comparison of the ventral epidural spreading in modified interlaminar approach and transforaminal approach: a randomized, double-blind study. Pain Med 2016;17:1620–7.

30. Sinofsky AH. Concordant provocation as a prognostic indicator during interlaminar lumbosacral epidural steroid injections. Pain Physician 2014;17:247–53.

31. Bogduk N. Lumbar transforaminal access. In: Bogduk N, editor. Practice guidelines for spinal diagnostic and treatment procedures. San Francisco (CA): International Spine Intervention Society; 2013. p. 552.

32. MacVicar J, King W, Landers MH, et al. The effectiveness of lumbar transforaminal injection of steroids: a comprehensive review with systematic analysis of the published data. Pain Med 2013;14(1):14–28.

33. Benny B, Azari P. The efficacy of lumbosacral transforaminal epidural steroid injections: a comprehensive literature review. J Back Musculoskelet Rehabil 2011; 24(2):67–76.

34. Roberts ST. Efficacy of lumbosacral transforaminal epidural steroid injections: a systematic review. PM R 2015;1(7):657–68.

35. Bogduk N. Lumbar transforaminal access. In: Bogduk N, editor. Practice guidelines for spinal diagnostic and treatment procedures. San Francisco (CA): International Spine Intervention Society; 2013. p. 465.

36. Smuck M. Incidence of simultaneous epidural and vascular injection during lumbosacral transforaminal epidural injections. Spine J 2007;7:79–82.

37. Furman MB. Injectate volumes needed to reach specific landmarks in lumbar transforaminal epidural injections. PM R 2010;2(7):625–35.

38. Chun EH. Effect of high-volume injectate in lumbar transforaminal epidural steroid injections: a randomized, active control trial. Pain Physician 2015;18:519–25.

39. Kambin P, Sampson S. Posterolateral percutaneous suction-excision of herniated lumbar intervertebral discs. Report of interim results. Clin Orthop Relat Res 1986; 207:37–43.

40. Park JW, Nam HS, Cho SK, et al. Kambin's triangle approach of lumbar transforaminal epidural injection with spinal stenosis. Ann Rehabil Med 2011;35(6): 833–43.
41. Murthy NS, Maus TP, Behrns CL. Intraforaminal location of the great anterior radiculomedullary artery (artery of Adamkiewicz): a retrospective review. Pain Med 2010;11:1756–64.
42. Levi D, Horn S. The incidence of intradiscal, intrathecal, and intravascular flow during the performance of retrodiscal (infraneural) approach for lumbar transforaminal epidural steroid injections. Pain Med 2016;17(8):1416–22.
43. Petrolla JJ, Furman MB. Lumbar transforaminal epidural steroid injection, infraneural approach. In: Furman MB, Lee TS, Berkwits L, editors. Atlas of image guided spinal procedures. 1st edition. Philadelphia: WB Saunders; 2013. p. 109.
44. Jasper JF. Lumbar retrodiscal transforaminal injection. Pain Physician 2007;10: 501–10.
45. Park KD, Lee JH, Park Y. Injectate volumes needed to reach specific landmarks and contrast pattern in Kambin's triangle approach with spinal stenosis. Ann Rehabil Med 2012;36(4):480–7.
46. Kim C, Choi HE, Kang S. Contrast spreading patterns in retrodiscal transforaminal epidural steroid injection. Ann Rehabil Med 2012;36(4):474–9.
47. Bogduk N. Lumbar transforaminal access. In: Bogduk N, editor. Practice guidelines for spinal diagnostic and treatment procedures. San Francisco (CA): International Spine Intervention Society; 2013. p. 472–5.
48. Furman MB, Butler SP, Kim RE, et al. Injectate volumes needed to reach specific landmarks in S1 transforaminal epidural injections. Pain Med 2012;13:1265–74.
49. Fish DE. The S1 "Scotty Dog": report of a technique for S1 transforaminal epidural steroid injection. Arch Phys Med Rehabil 2007;88(12):1730–3.
50. El-Yahchouchi CA. Lumbar transforaminal epidural steroid injections: does immediate post-procedure pain response predict longer term effectiveness? Pain Med 2014;15(6):921–8.
51. Singla A. Preoperative lumbar epidural injections are associated with increased risk of infection after single level lumbar decompression: a nationwide database analysis of 62,241 cases. Spine J 2015;15(10):S126.
52. El-Yahchouchi CA. Adverse event rates associated with transforaminal and interlaminar epidural steroid injections: a multi-institutional study. Pain Med 2016; 17(2):239–47.
53. Plastaras C. Adverse events associated with fluoroscopically guided lumbosacral transforaminal epidural steroid injections. Spine J 2015;15(10):2157–65.
54. Horlocker TT, Wedel DJ, Schroeder DR, et al. Preoperative antiplatelet therapy does not increase the risk of spinal hematoma associated with regional anesthesia. Anesth Analg 1995;80:303–9.
55. Horlocker TT, Bajwa ZH, Ashraf Z, et al. Risk assessment of hemorrhagic complications associated with nonsteroidal anti-inflammatory medications in ambulatory pain clinic patients undergoing epidural steroid injection. Anesth Analg 2002;95: 1691–7.
56. Enders S. The risks of continuing or discontinuing anticoagulants for patients undergoing common interventional pain procedures. Pain Med 2017;18:403–9.
57. Goodman BS, House LM, Vallabhaneni S, et al. Anticoagulant and antiplatelet management for spinal procedures: a prospective, descriptive study and interpretation of guidelines. Pain Med 2017;18(7):1218–24.

Ultrasound-Guided Interventions of the Cervical Spine and Nerves

Ke-Vin Chang, MD, PhD[a], Wei-Ting Wu, MD[a],
Levent Özçakar, MD[b],*

KEYWORDS

- Neck • Pain • Ultrasound • Nerve • Injection

KEY POINTS

- The cervical region has a complicated neurovascular network and familiarization with the regional sonoanatomy is the basis before proceeding to ultrasound (US)-guided injections.
- The in-plane technique with visualization of the whole needle should be preferred for the injection of cervical nerves.
- Comprehensive understanding of the cervical sonoanatomy should remain as the prerequisite before one can plan US-guided cervical interventions.

INTRODUCTION

Because high resolution ultrasound (US) promptly depicts muscles, tendons, ligaments, and peripheral nerves, it is among the best imaging modalities for guiding perineural injections.[1–8] Cervical sonoanatomy is actually quite complicated and several years of scanning experience on the extremities is required before practicing US-guided injections on the neck.[8–11] Additionally, awareness of the sonographic appearance and location of the vital structures (eg, trachea, carotid artery, vertebral artery, vagus nerve, and spinal cord) can significantly reduce the chance of collateral injury.[8] Although there are numerous US-guided regimens or techniques; that is, local anesthetics, corticosteroids, dextrose, platelet-rich plasma, and radiofrequency ablation, their effectiveness still heavily relies on the precision of the intervention. Although the comparison of efficacy among various injectates is not within the scope of this

Disclosure: The authors have nothing to disclose.
[a] Department of Physical Medicine and Rehabilitation, National Taiwan University Hospital, Bei-Hu Branch and National Taiwan University College of Medicine, 87 Neijiang Street, Wanhua, Taipei City 108, Taiwan; [b] Department of Physical and Rehabilitation Medicine, Hacettepe University Medical School, Hacettepe Üniversitesi Tıp Fakültesi Hastaneleri Zemin Kat FTR AD, Sıhhıye, Ankara 06100, Turkey
* Corresponding author.
E-mail address: lozcakar@yahoo.com

Phys Med Rehabil Clin N Am 29 (2018) 93–103
https://doi.org/10.1016/j.pmr.2017.08.008
1047-9651/18/© 2017 Elsevier Inc. All rights reserved.

article, the risk of thrombosis due to intravascular administration of crystalloid cortico-steroids is noteworthy in regard to cervical interventions.[12] Overall, the purpose of this article is to deliberate the sonoanatomy of the commonly intervened cervical structures and to illustrate how those procedures can safely and precisely be performed under US-guidance.

Selective Cervical Root Block

Indication
The selective cervical root block procedure is usually necessary in patients with cervical radiculopathy in association with a herniated disc or an osseous foraminal encroachment.[13]

Anatomy
The brachial plexus is composed of the ventral rami from the 5th cervical nerve (C) to the 1st thoracic nerve (T), and is divided into roots, trunks, divisions, cords, and peripheral nerves. The superior trunk is made of C5 and C6 nerve roots, C7 continues as the middle trunk, and C8 and T1 roots form the inferior trunk. Each trunk is then divided into the anterior and posterior divisions. The lateral cord receives nerve fibers from the anterior divisions of the superior and middle trunks, the medial cord is derived from the anterior division of the inferior trunk, and all the 3 posterior divisions merge to continue as the posterior cord. The lateral cord gives off the musculocutaneous and lateral pectoral nerves; the medial cord gives off the ulnar, medial pectoral, and medial cutaneous nerves of the upper limb; and the posterior cord gives off the upper and lower subscapular nerves, thoracodorsal, radial, and axillary nerves. The median nerve obtains its innervation from the medial and lateral cords.[8]

Sonoanatomy and technique
The patient is positioned supine with the head rotating to the contralateral side. The transducer is first placed on the supraclavicular fossa in the sagittal plane where the subclavian vessels and supraclavicular portion of the brachial plexus can be visualized. At this localization, the brachial plexus looks like grapes or a cluster of hypoechoic round structures, located dorsal and superior to the subclavian artery. Relocating the transducer more cranially, the brachial plexus can be followed in the interscalene region where the cervical nerve roots are arranged in a line between the anterior and medial scalene muscles. At this level, the most superficial is the C5 nerve root and the deepest is the T1 nerve root.[8]

Moving the transducer toward the head, the C7 transverse process can easily be recognized as having only 1 prominent posterior tubercle. Yet, its configuration is different from those of C3-C6, all of which have anterior and posterior tubercles. Because the vertebral artery enters the transverse foramina at the level of C6 in most people, the course of the artery can be confirmed at the level of C7 by using power Doppler US imaging. Herein, the short axis of the C7 nerve root can be visualized anterior to the C7 transverse process and posterior to the vertebral artery.[8] Further advancing the transducer more cranially, the C6 nerve root is seen emerging from the intertubercular groove, bordered by the anterior and posterior tubercles of the transverse process. The anterior tubercle of the C6 transverse process, also known as Chassaignac tubercle, is prominent in most people and is usually longer than the posterior tubercle of the same level. The C5 nerve root can be tracked by using the same approach.[8]

The patient is supine with the head rotated to the contralateral side and the injection is performed from lateral to medial using the in-plane approach (**Fig. 1**A). The needle can be introduced selectively at C5 (**Fig. 1**B), C6 (**Fig. 1**C), and C7 (**Fig. 1**D) levels until

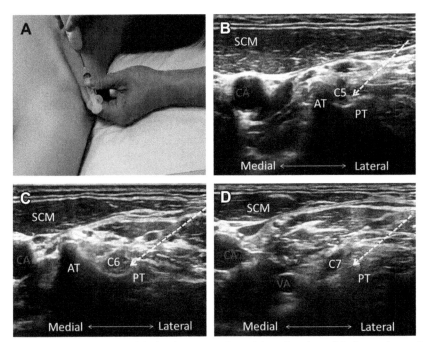

Fig. 1. Selective cervical root block. The patient is positioned supine with the neck rotating to the contralateral side (*A*) and the transducer is placed horizontally while the needle (*yellow arrow*) is inserted from lateral to medial, targeting the C5 (*B*), C6 (*C*), and C7 (*D*) nerve roots. AT, anterior tubercle of the transverse process; CA, carotid artery; PT, posterior tubercle of the transverse process; SCM, sternocleidomastoid; VA, vertebral artery.

the anterior border of the posterior tubercle of the C7 transverse process. It is noteworthy that dorsal scapular and long thoracic nerves emerge from the root level of the brachial plexus and should be avoided while advancing the needle.[8,14]

Superficial Cervical Plexus Block

Indication
The superficial cervical plexus block procedure is indicated for patients who are planned to undergo carotid endarterectomy and superficial neck surgeries, or those with ear and neck pain caused by entrapment of the superficial cervical plexus.[15]

Anatomy
The superficial cervical plexus, originating from C1-C4 roots, innervates the skin on the lateral aspect of the neck and the supraclavicular region. It comprises the lesser occipital, greater auricular, transverse cervical, and supraclavicular nerves.[8]

Sonoanatomy and technique
The patient is positioned supine with the neck rotated to the contralateral side. The needle is introduced from lateral to medial though the in-plane approach (**Fig. 2A**). The transducer is placed axially at the level of C4 vertebra, which is also approximately at the same level of the thyroid cartilage. The superficial cervical plexus, appearing as a group of several hypoechoic round structures, is interposed between the sternoclei-domastoid muscle superficially and the anterior or middle scalene and levator scapulae muscles deeply (**Fig. 2B**). The procedure should be avoided in patients with

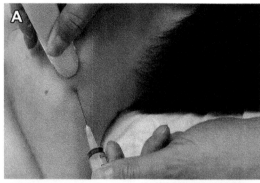

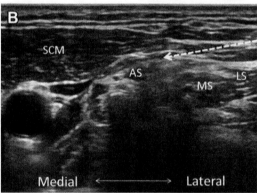

Fig. 2. Superficial cervical plexus block. The patient is positioned supine with the neck rotating to the contralateral side (*A*) and the transducer is placed horizontally while the needle (*yellow arrow*) is inserted from lateral to medial, targeting the facial plane between the SCM muscle superficially and the AS, MS, and LS muscles deeply (*B*). AS, anterior scalene muscle; LS, levator scapulae muscle; MS, middle scalene muscle.

preexisting respiratory disorders because local anesthetics may occasionally be distributed more anteriorly, causing phrenic nerve paralysis.[16]

Stellate Ganglion Block

Indication
The stellate ganglion block procedure is indicated for patients with various painful syndromes of the head, neck, and upper limbs due to dysregulated sympathetic nerve activity.[17]

Anatomy
The stellate (or cervicothoracic) ganglion is part of the sympathetic chain formed by the inferior cervical and first thoracic ganglia. It lies anterior to the C7 transverse process and the neck of the first rib. It is situated between the prevertebral fascia and longus coli muscles, and provides efferent sympathetic signals to the head, neck, heart, and upper extremities.[17]

Sonoanatomy and technique
The patient is positioned supine with the neck rotating to the contralateral side (**Fig. 3**A). The transducer is placed axially at the anterolateral aspect of the neck

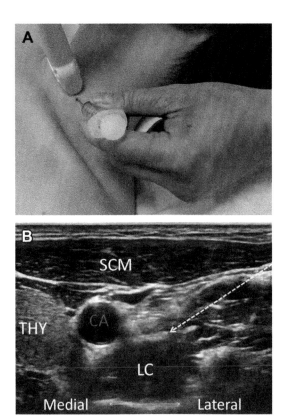

Fig. 3. Stellate ganglion block. The patient is positioned supine with the neck rotating to the contralateral side (*A*) and the transducer is placed horizontally while the needle (*yellow arrow*) is inserted from lateral to medial, targeting the prevertebral fascia anterior to the longus coli (LC) muscle (*B*). THY, thyroid gland.

and then moved cranially and caudally to recognize C6 and C7 vertebrae (using the aforementioned approach). The muscle is located medial to the Chassaignac tubercle and the vertebral body is beside the longus coli muscle. The needle is introduced from lateral to medial though the window posterior to the carotid neurovascular bundle using the in-plane approach (**Fig. 3**B). The target is the area deep to the prevertebral fascia but superficial to the longus coli muscle. Because the procedure is not performed exactly at the C7-T1 level, cervical sympathetic chain block would be a better terminology for this technique. The power Doppler mode should be switched on before injection to prevent injury of the inferior thyroid, vertebral, and carotid arteries.[17]

Cervical Medial Branch Block

Indication
The cervical medial branch block procedure is indicated for patients with painful conditions due to involvement of the cervical facet joints.[18]

Anatomy
After the cervical nerve roots exit from the intervertebral foramina, they give off the ventral and dorsal rami. The latter are then divided into the medial and lateral branches. The dorsal ramus of the first cervical nerve innervates the suboccipital

muscles and does not have a clearly defined medial branch. The medial branch of the second cervical nerve is the greater occipital nerve (GON), which supplies the posterior scalp and the semispinalis capitis muscle. The third cervical nerve has a superficial and a deep medial branch; the superficial nerve is also known as the third occipital nerve (TON). The deep medial branch of the third cervical nerve and the medial branches of C4-C6 nerves are more typical, coursing around the articular pillars to provide sensation to the facet joints. These joints receive dual innervation from the medial branches of the adjacent 2 vertebral levels. For example, the C4-C5 facet joint is innervated by the medial branches of C4-C5 nerve roots. An important point regarding the bony anatomy of the articular pillars is that they end at the second cervical level. The atlantooccipital (C1-C0) and atlantoaxial (C1-C2) joints are located anterior to the articular pillars.[8]

Sonoanatomy and technique
A side-lying position exposing the lateral neck is preferred. The transducer is placed along the long axis, starting from the mastoid process of the temporal bone. The prominent transverse process of the C1 vertebra is seen as a small hyperechoic curved plane, whereas the atlantooccipital joint is located deeply between the C1 transverse process and the mastoid process.

The transducer is then shifted posterior and caudal. The inferior articular process of C2 is seen as an oblique bony cliff, connecting to the C3 superior articular process. Sonographic image of the lateral aspect of the cervical articular pillars appears wavy where each peak of the waves represents the facet joints. The medial branches usually course though the valleys of the wavy appearance. The only exception is the

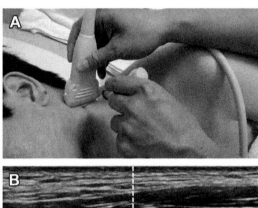
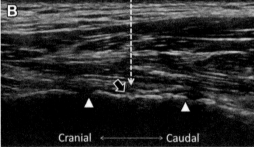

Fig. 4. Cervical medial branch block using the out-of-plane approach. The patient is positioned side-lying and the transducer is placed along the long axis of the lateral neck (A). The needle (yellow arrow) is introduced from anterior to posterior, targeting the short axis of the cervical medial branch (black arrow), which lies between the cervical facet joints of 2 adjacent levels (white arrowheads) (B).

C7 medial branch, which passes around the junction between the superior articular process of C7 and the base of the transverse process.

One injection technique may be through the out-of-plane approach while the transducer is aligned parallel to the long-axis of the articular pillars. The needle is introduced anteroposteriorly (**Fig. 4**A), targeting the short axis of the medial branch which appears as a hypoechoic round structure (**Fig. 4**B). With this technique, insertion of the needle from posterior to anterior is prohibited due to the high risk of erroneous direction of the needle into the intervertebral foramen causing spinal cord injury.[19,20]

An alternative method is the in-plane approach, targeting the long axis of the medial branch by redirecting the transducer along the axial plane (**Fig. 5**). This technique allows the full visualization of the needle tract and reduces the collateral injury of the adjacent neurovascular structures. The use of power Doppler is suggested to locate the radicular arteries before injection because those vessels may masquerade as medial branches in gray scale imaging.

Greater Occipital Nerve Block

Indication
The GON block procedure is indicated for patients with occipital neuralgia due to entrapment of the GON.[21]

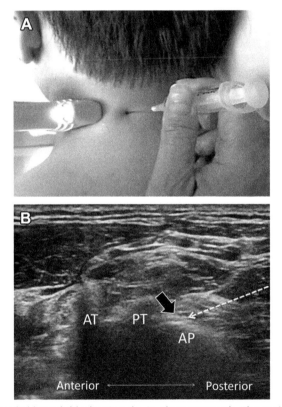

Fig. 5. Cervical medial branch block using the in-plane approach. The patient is positioned prone and the transducer is placed horizontally on the lateral neck (*A*). The needle (*yellow arrow*) is introduced from posterior to anterior, targeting the long axis of the cervical medial branch (*black arrow*) (*B*). AP, articular pillar.

Anatomy

The GON is the medial branch of the second cervical nerve. After being diverged from the dorsal ramus, it wraps the inferior border of the inferior obliquus capitis muscle and courses medially and cranially under the semispinalis capitis muscle. It then pierces the semispinalis capitis and trapezius muscles and reaches the posterior region of the scalp. When the nerve becomes superficial just below the superior nuchal line, it runs between the occipital artery laterally and the occipital protuberance medially.[8]

Sonoanatomy and technique

The patient is positioned prone, bending the neck ventrally (**Fig. 6A**). The transducer is first placed axially above the superior nuchal line and then relocated caudally. The posterior ring of the atlas is seen as a hyperechoic semicircular structure. Moving the transducer more caudally, spinous process of the second cervical vertebra (usually bifid) is visualized with the laminae at both sides extending like bird wings. As the lateral edge of the transducer is further pivoted cranially and laterally, the

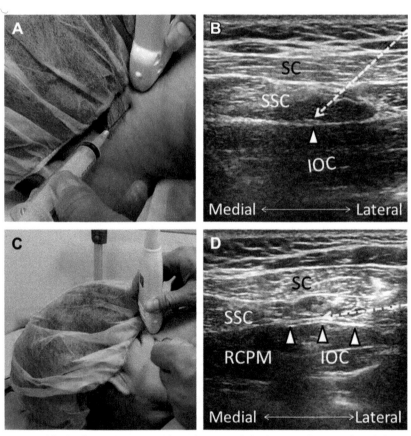

Fig. 6. GON block. The patient is positioned prone while the transducer is placed along the long axis of the obliquus capitis inferior muscle (*A*). The needle (*yellow arrows*) is introduced from lateral to medial, targeting the greater occipital nerve (*white arrowheads*) in its short axis (*B*). The transducer is redirected to align with the short axis of the obliquus capitis inferior muscle (*C*) and the needle is introduced from lateral to medial, targeting the greater occipital nerve in its long axis (*D*). IOC, inferior obliquus capitis; RCPM, rectus capitis posterior major; SC, splenius capitis; SSC, semispinalis capitis.

wedge-shaped huge muscle (inferior obliquus capitis) is visualized between the C2 spinous process and C1 transverse process. The short axis of the GON is seen as a hypoechoic dot located between this muscle deeply and the semispinalis capitis muscle superficially.

The needle is introduced from lateral to medial until the nerve is reached (**Fig. 6**B). Compared with the medial to lateral approach, this approach can avoid piercing the tough trapezius fascia, which might easily divert the needle superficially. The transducer can also be aligned parallel to the long axis of the GON for hydrodissection of its whole course (**Fig. 6**C,D).

The Third Occipital Nerve

Indication
The TON procedure is indicated for patients with occipital headache referred from the C2-C3 facet joint.[22]

Anatomy
The TON is the superficial medial branch of the third cervical nerve. After branching from the dorsal ramus, the nerve wraps around the C2-C3 facet joint and courses cranially and dorsally into the same facial plane containing the GON. It runs parallel and medial to the GON in the midline of the posterior neck and innervates the posterior middle scalp.[8]

Sonoanatomy and technique
The patient lies on the side and the transducer is placed along the long axis of the lateral neck where the articular pillars, wavy continuous structures, are seen (**Fig. 7**A). The transducer is moved to the most cranial portion until the top of the

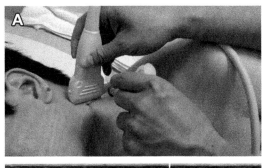

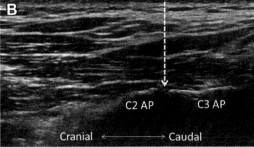

Fig. 7. TON block. The patient is positioned side-lying and the transducer is placed along the long axis of the lateral neck (*A*). The needle (*yellow arrow*) is introduced from anterior to posterior, targeting the short axis of the TON (*B*).

articular pillar, the inferior articular process of the second cervical vertebra, is visualized. The bony gap between the C2 inferior articular process and the C3 superior articular process is the C2-C3 facet joint. In the short axis, the TON appears as a hypoechoic circular structure located above or near the C2-C3 facet joint.

Similar to the cervical medial branch block, an out-of-plane approach, directing the needle from anterior to posterior, can be used (**Fig. 7**B). The power Doppler imaging of the target region should be examined ahead of the injection to prevent accidental injuries to the vertebral, radicular, or deep cervical arteries.

SUMMARY

Comprehensive understanding of the cervical sonoanatomy should remain as the prerequisite before one can plan US-guided cervical interventions. Certainly, the in-plane technique, during which visualization of the whole needle tract is possible, is safer and more comfortable for the physician. Appropriate use of the power Doppler mode is highly recommended to locate the adjacent critical vessels before the intervention. Last but not least, planning how to properly position the patient and plot the route to reach the target is crucial but might be more time-consuming then the injection itself.

REFERENCES

1. Özçakar L, Kara M, Chang KV, et al. EURO-MUSCULUS/USPRM basic scanning protocols for wrist and hand. Eur J Phys Rehabil Med 2015;51:479–84.
2. Özçakar L, Kara M, Chang KV, et al. EURO-MUSCULUS/USPRM basic scanning protocols for knee. Eur J Phys Rehabil Med 2015;51:641–6.
3. Özçakar L, Kara M, Chang KV, et al. EURO-MUSCULUS/USPRM basic scanning protocols for shoulder. Eur J Phys Rehabil Med 2015;51:491–6.
4. Özçakar L, Kara M, Chang KV, et al. EURO-MUSCULUS/USPRM basic scanning protocols for elbow. Eur J Phys Rehabil Med 2015;51:485–9.
5. Özçakar L, Kara M, Chang KV, et al. Nineteen reasons why physiatrists should do musculoskeletal ultrasound: EURO-MUSCULUS/USPRM recommendations. Am J Phys Med Rehabil 2015;94:e45–9.
6. Özçakar L, Kara M, Chang KV, et al. EURO-MUSCULUS/USPRM basic scanning protocols for ankle and foot. Eur J Phys Rehabil Med 2015;51:647–53.
7. Özçakar L, Kara M, Chang KV, et al. EURO-MUSCULUS/USPRM basic scanning protocols for hip. Eur J Phys Rehabil Med 2015;51:635–40.
8. Chang KV, Lin CP, Hung CY, et al. Sonographic nerve tracking in the cervical region: a pictorial essay and video demonstration. Am J Phys Med Rehabil 2016; 95:862–70.
9. Hung CY, Hsiao MY, Özçakar L, et al. Sonographic tracking of the lower limb peripheral nerves: a pictorial essay and video demonstration. Am J Phys Med Rehabil 2016;95:698–708.
10. Wu CH, Chang KV, Özcakar L, et al. Sonographic tracking of the upper limb peripheral nerves: a pictorial essay and video demonstration. Am J Phys Med Rehabil 2015;94:740–7.
11. Chang KV, Lin CP, Lin CS, et al. Sonographic tracking of trunk nerves: essential for ultrasound-guided pain management and research. J Pain Res 2017;10: 79–88.
12. Epstein NE. The risks of epidural and transforaminal steroid injections in the spine: commentary and a comprehensive review of the literature. Surg Neurol Int 2013;4(Suppl 2):S74–93.

13. Huston CW, Slipman CW. Diagnostic selective nerve root blocks: indications and usefulness. Phys Med Rehabil Clin N Am 2002;13:545–65.
14. Narouze SN, Vydyanathan A, Kapural L, et al. Ultrasound-guided cervical selective nerve root block: a fluoroscopy-controlled feasibility study. Reg Anesth Pain Med 2009;34:343–8.
15. Pandit JJ, Satya-Krishna R, Gration P. Superficial or deep cervical plexus block for carotid endarterectomy: a systematic review of complications. Br J Anaesth 2007;99:159–69.
16. Herring AA, Stone MB, Frenkel O, et al. The ultrasound-guided superficial cervical plexus block for anesthesia and analgesia in emergency care settings. Am J Emerg Med 2012;30:1263–7.
17. Narouze S. Ultrasound-guided stellate ganglion block: safety and efficacy. Curr Pain Headache Rep 2014;18:424.
18. Manchikanti L, Singh V, Falco FJ, et al. Comparative outcomes of a 2-year follow-up of cervical medial branch blocks in management of chronic neck pain: a randomized, double-blind controlled trial. Pain Physician 2010;13:437–50.
19. Chang KV, Wu WT, Özçakar L. Ultrasound-guided C7 cervical medial branch block using the in-plane approach. Am J Phys Med Rehabil 2017;96(9):e164.
20. Park D, Seong MY, Kim HY, et al. Spinal cord injury during ultrasound-guided C7 cervical medial branch block. Am J Phys Med Rehabil 2017;96(6):e111–4.
21. Shim JH, Ko SY, Bang MR, et al. Ultrasound-guided greater occipital nerve block for patients with occipital headache and short term follow up. Korean J Anesthesiol 2011;61:50–4.
22. Lord SM, Barnsley L, Wallis BJ, et al. Third occipital nerve headache: a prevalence study. J Neurol Neurosurg Psychiatry 1994;57:1187–90.

Sonographic Guide for Botulinum Toxin Injections of the Neck Muscles in Cervical Dystonia

CrossMark

Bayram Kaymak, MD[a], Murat Kara, MD[a], Eda Gürçay, MD[b], Levent Özçakar, MD[a],*

KEYWORDS

- Cervical dystonia • Muscle • Ultrasound • Botulinum toxin • Innervation zone

KEY POINTS

- Intramuscular botulinum toxin (BoTX) injection is the first-line treatment of cervical dystonia.
- In addition to its considerable benefits, poor treatment outcomes and some side effects have also been reported after BoTX applications.
- One of the most important reasons is incorrect localization of the needle during toxin injections.
- Although electromyography has commonly been used to detect targeted and dystonic muscles, without imaging, it is impossible to truly verify precise needle positioning in the proper muscle.
- Ultrasound has been recommended because of its high capability in illustrating most of the neck muscles.

INTRODUCTION

Cervical dystonia (CD) is the most commonly seen focal primary dystonia, characterized by involuntary contractions of the neck muscles resulting in abnormal movements and posture of the head and neck. Intramuscular botulinum toxin (BoTX) injection is the first-line treatment and several studies have reported its benefit in reducing dystonia and associated symptoms (eg, pain).[1-3] Poor treatment outcomes, weakness of uninjected muscles, and some side effects, however, such as dysphagia, dysphonia, dry mouth, and ptosis, have also been reported after toxin injections.[2,4-8] The 2 likely/considerable reasons are inaccurate detection of the dystonic muscles and imprecise

The authors have nothing to disclose.
a Department of Physical and Rehabilitation Medicine, Hacettepe University Medical School, Ankara 06100, Turkey; b Department of Physical and Rehabilitation Medicine, Gaziler Training and Research Hospital, Lodumlu yolu, 06800 Bilkent, Ankara, Turkey
* Corresponding author. Hacettepe Üniversitesi, Tıp Fakültesi, Hastaneleri Zemin Kat FTR AD, Sıhhıye, Ankara 06100, Turkey.
E-mail address: lozcakar@yahoo.com

Phys Med Rehabil Clin N Am 29 (2018) 105–123
https://doi.org/10.1016/j.pmr.2017.08.009

injections.[5,9] Electromyography (EMG) has commonly been used for detecting the dystonic muscles or targeting the proper muscles for BoTX injections in CD patients.[10,11] Physicians cannot truly verify, however, that the needle is located in the targeted muscle without imaging guidance, for example, ultrasound (US).[9,12] In addition to incorrect needle placement, the aforementioned side effects have also been attributed to the spread of BoTX into the adjacent structures.[13,14] Furthermore, anatomic variations, obesity, abnormal neck and head posture, and atrophy of the neck muscles may also increase the risk of incorrect needle placement using EMG or palpation guidance.[12,15–18] In 1 study, it was observed that although dysphagia ensued as a complication after EMG-guided injections, it was not encountered when US guidance was added thereafter.[9]

Neck muscles are small and thin and some have complex orientation compared with extremity muscles. Additionally, several vital neurovascular structures pass through the head/neck and thorax in close proximity with these muscles. Therefore, imaging guidance is highly recommended.[4] Furthermore, in clinical practice, due to the difficulties in localizing/accessing them, deep cervical muscles are generally not injected. Desirable clinical improvement cannot be achieved without injecting those deep muscles, which are frequently involved in complex forms of CD.[19] In this regard, because almost all of the neck muscles can precisely be scanned with US imaging, accurate assignment of dystonic activity to a specific muscle during EMG evaluations and distribution of the toxin within the targeted muscle during injections can be ensured.[12] US is convenient and patient/physician friendly and provides real-time imaging without radiation exposure.[20] Its use in musculoskeletal practice has been widely accepted and already standardized.[21–27]

Innervation zone (IZ)–targeted BoTX injections are found to be more effective with less side effects compared with nontargeted applications. In this sense, US guidance is recommended while performing BoTX injections to IZs of different compartments in a muscle. Besides, the best treatment outcomes are received with lower toxin doses.[12,28–31] US may also be used to detect morphologic and architectural features of the skeletal muscles, which determine the functional properties, distribution of IZs, and the spreading of BoTX.[29] **Fig. 1** provides an example of compartmentalization of the sternocleidomastoid muscle (SCM) in a healthy subject.

Overall, morphologic/architectural features, IZs, and proper sites for BoTX injection of neck muscles, which are commonly injected in patients with CD, are summarized in this review article. The figures are arranged so as to display the probe positionings, relevant schematic drawings in the axial plane, and the corresponding US images. Muscle selection or clinical features of CD are not within the scope of this review.

MORPHOLOGY AND ARCHITECTURE OF NECK MUSCLES

Movements of the head and cervical joints are performed by approximately 20 neck muscles, some of which are commonly affected in CD (**Table 1**).[2,32] Morphologic (origin, insertion, shape, and compartments) and architectural (fascicle length, pennation angle, and cross-sectional area [CSA]) features of the neck muscles determine their function, distribution of the IZs, and the spread of BoTX.[29] Neuromuscular junctions (NMJs) of a muscle may be clustered in 1 or more 3-D arranged bandlike regions called IZs or scattered throughout the muscle volume.

Because there is a paucity of data regarding the IZs of the neck muscles, in most of them, the authors tried to deduce the IZs based on the morphologic and architectural features of each muscle. Using US and high-quality cross-sectional photographs of a fresh cadaver, it was generally assumed that the IZs are located in the bulkiest region

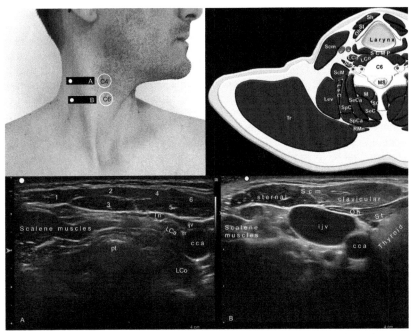

Fig. 1. When the probe is positioned in the axial plane at C4 (A) and C6 (B) levels, SCM and its compartments (1-6) can be seen in details. cca, common carotid artery; ijv, internal jugular vein; LCa, longus capitis; LCo, longus colli; ln, lymph node; Lev, levator scapulae; LsC, longissimus cervicis; MS, medulla spinalis; n, vagal nerve; Oh, omohyoid; pt, posterior tubercle; RMn, rhomboid minor; SC, spinalis cervicis; ScA, scalenus anterior; ScM, scalenus medius; Scm, sternocleidomastoid; SCMP, superior constrictor muscle of pharynx; SeCa, semispinalis capitis; Sh, sternohyoid; St, sternothyroid; SpC, splenius cervicis; SpCa, splenius capitis; Tr, trapezius..

of the targeted muscle. It was also assumed that a neck muscle has 1 IZ passing through the middle of the fascicles, if it does not have any inscription and is composed of fascicles whose lengths are less than 130 mm.[29,33] In CD patients with severe dystonic posture, the authors recommend finding the injection points using US rather than the anatomic landmarks because, due the dystonic activity of the muscles, the normal anatomic relationship between the landmarks might easily be deteriorated. Number of injection sites was recommended according to the fascicle length and the number/

Table 1
Commonly affected muscles in cervical dystonia

Anterior	Lateral	Posterior
SCM	Scalenus anterior	Trapezius
Longus colli	Scalenus medius	Levator scapulae
Longus capitis	Scalenus posterior	Splenius capitis/splenius cervicis
Rectus capitis anterior	Rectus capitis lateralis	Semispinalis capitis/cervicis Longissimus capitis/cervicis Obliquus capitis superior/inferior Rectus capitis posterior major/minor

size of the IZs, which are correlated with compartmentalization, 3-D muscle fiber arrangement, and CSA of the muscle.

Spreading of the BoTX in the muscle tissue is also important.[29] In a spastic human muscle, it was detected 3.2 cm along and 0.7 cm perpendicular to the fascicles.[34] Therefore, in thick and wide muscles, BoTX injection should be applied into 2 or more points perpendicular (vertically or horizontally) to muscle fascicles, or the needle should be moved along the line perpendicular to muscle fascicles during the procedure. Injections should be applied in the midportion of the muscle belly at recommended points, to ensure homogenous distribution, which is possible only with US guidance. Lastly, physiologic CSA (PCSA), muscle length and pennation angle, which are proportional to muscle strength and excursion may be useful to decide on the dosage of BoTX for individual muscles.

ANTERIOR NECK
Sternocleidomastoid

- The SCM is a wide and thin muscle. It has 2 heads (sternal and clavicular) and 5 anatomic compartments (3 superficial and 2 deep) with different attachment sites.[32,35] Although the sternal head shows a rounded shape, the clavicular head has a flat shape. Sternooccipital, cleido-occipital, and superficial parts of the sternomastoid compartments elongate parallel to each other and form the superficial sheet of the SCM (see **Fig. 1**). Sterno-occipital and superficial parts of the sternomastoid compartments are not visibly and sonographically separable from each other.[35] Cleidomastoid and deep parts of the sternomastoid compartments form the deep anatomic compartment. SCM has a wide range of variations.[36,37] In **Fig. 1**, an extraclavicular head is illustrated. Regarding volume and PCSA, sternomastoid compartments (superficial and deep) are largest, followed by cleidomastoid and sternooccipital compartments that have approximately equal values. The cleidooccipital compartment is the smallest one.[32,35]
  - In an animal study, SCM was found to have 5 compartments similar to human SCM. It was also stated that SCM is divided into 2 functional compartments (superficial and deep) according to muscle fiber type. Investigators have suggested that the superficial compartment, including mostly type 2 myofibers, may be responsible for the rapid movement of the head. The deep compartment, composed of both type 1 and type 2 myofibers, may act to maintain the head posture.[38] To the authors' knowledge, clinical significance of anatomic and functional compartmentalization of SCM has not been explored yet.
- Dystonic involvement of different compartments may also differ from each other, because neuromuscular compartments in a muscle are innervated by distinct neuronal pools.[39] Therefore, BoTX injection may also be targeted to specific compartments of SCM when treating CD. In all compartments, fascicles elongate through the length of the muscle belly without being interrupted by any tendinous inscription. The range of fascicle length is 7.0 cm to 15.5 cm in SCM[35] and this indicates that SCM does not include serially connected compartments.
- The IZs of SCM were investigated with acetylcholinesterase staining in an animal study[38] whereby their number was observed to change according the muscle length. The distance between the IZs had the range of 1 cm to 3 cm. In accordance with these results, Lee and colleagues[40] detected that

intramuscular motor points of human SCM are densely located at 20% to 70% of the distance between the mastoid and the most medial portion of the clavicle. Density of intramuscular motor points per length was also illustrated in that study. IZs of SCM were also studied using superficial EMG and found located around the midpoint or the lower border of the superior one-third of the muscle.[28,41] Surface EMG has some limitations, however, in evaluating the whole distribution of the IZs in skeletal muscles. Yet, deep compartments cannot be evaluated.[29]

- The authors' recommendation for the injection sites are the levels 30% and 60% of the distance between the mastoid and the most medial portion of the clavicle. Depending on the width of the muscle, injections should be applied at these levels in 1 or 2 points, which are located on a line perpendicular to fascicle alignment with a distance of 2 cm in between.

Longus Capitis

- The longus capitis muscle has 2 heads (or anatomic compartments). The short head (located superomedially) comprises fascicles originating from C2 and C3 transverse processes and inserting to the basilar part of the occipital bone. The long head (located more laterally) originates from the transverse processes of C4-C6 vertebrae and attaches to the aponeurosis covering the surface. Lengths of the fascicles arising from the lower cervical vertebrae are longer than upper ones and change between 1.2 cm and 7.7 cm. PCSA of longus capitis is 0.92 cm^2.[32] Although data could not be found concerning the functional compartmentalization, the authors believe that the superomedial head attaching to the occipital bone may have dominant effects on head movements. There are no data regarding the IZs of the longus capitis muscles either.
- Ideally BoTX injection should be performed at 2 points, superomedial and inferolateral compartments. Because injection for the former may be technically difficult, the authors recommend that BoTX injection for longus capitis should be performed at 1 point at the level of C3 vertebra (**Fig. 2**).

Longus Colli

- Longus colli lays on the anterior surface of the C1-T3 vertebrae. It is divided into 3 parts (anatomic compartments). Superior oblique part originates from the anterior tubercles of the transverse processes of C3-C5 vertebrae and runs superomedially to attach on the tubercle on the anterior arch of atlas. Vertical intermediate part arises from the anterior aspect of C5-T3 vertebral bodies, ascends superiorly, and attaches to the anterior aspect of the C2-4 vertebrae. Inferior oblique (the smallest) part originates from the T1-T2 or T3 vertebrae and runs superolaterally and attaches to the anterior tubercles of the transverse processes of C5-C6 vertebrae.[32]
- The authors could not find any data about the IZs and functional compartmentalization of longus colli. Its anatomic compartments may have distinct functions on the neck. Oblique parts may flex the neck laterally and inferior oblique part rotates the neck to the opposite side.[42] These may be taken into account when evaluating patients with CD and applying BoTX injections.
- The authors recommend that the injection should be performed at 2 points at the levels of C3 and C6 vertebrae (see **Fig. 2**).

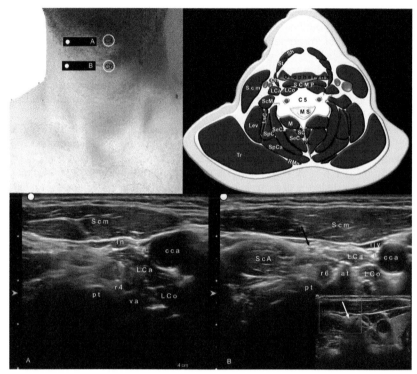

Fig. 2. When the probe is positioned in the axial plane at C4 (A) and C6 (B) levels, longus capitis and longus colli muscles can be seen. Branch of the thyrocervical trunk *(black arrow)* is visualized in B-mode (B) and power Doppler *(inlet)* images. White arrow indicates the phrenic nerve. at, anterior tubercle; cca, common carotid artery; ijv, internal jugular vein; LCo, longus colli; Lev, levator scapulae; ln, lymph node; LsC, longissimus cervicis; M, multifidus; MS, medulla spinalis; n, vagal nerve; NL, nuchal ligament; Oh, omohyoid; r4, fourth nerve root; r6, sixth nerve root; RMn, rhomboid minor; pt, posterior tubercle; SC, spinalis cervicis; ScA, scalenus anterior; ScM, scalenus medius; Scm, sternocleidomastoid; SCMP, superior constrictor muscle of pharynx; SeC, semispinalis cervicis; SeCa, semispinalis capitis; Sh, sternohyoid; St, sternothyroid; SpC, splenius cervicis; SpCa, splenius capitis; Tr, trapezius; va, vertebral artery.

LATERAL NECK
Scalenus Anterior

- Fascicles of scalenus anterior insert on the anterior tubercles of the transverse processes of C3-C6 vertebrae. While descending, they converge, blend, and attach to the scalene tubercle on the first rib.
- Length of the fascicles ranges between 3.3 cm and 6.3 cm and the CSA of scalenus anterior muscle is 1.45 cm^2.[32]
- There are no data about the functional compartmentalization of scalenus anterior. Its IZ was investigated in a study. It has been shown that the IZs reside around the midpoint or in the superior portion of the muscle.[41]
- The authors recommend that BoTX injection for scalenus anterior should be performed at 1 point at the level of C7-T1 vertebrae (**Fig. 3**).

Scalenus Medius

- Fascicles of scalenus medius attach to the transverse processes of axis and the posterior tubercle of the transverse processes of C3-C7 vertebrae. Distally, the

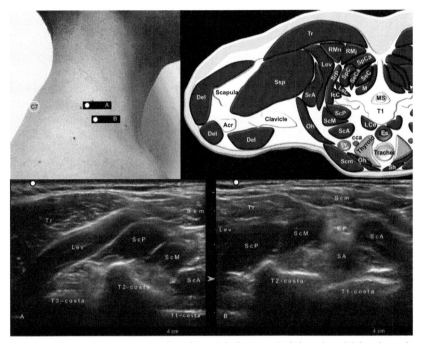

Fig. 3. When the probe is positioned in the axial plane at C7 (A) and T1 (B) levels, scalenus anterior, medius, posterior, and levator scapulae muscles are seen. Acr, acromion; BP, brachial plexus; cca, common carotid artery; Cor, coracoid process; Del, deltoid; Es, esophagus; H, humerus; IcC, iliocostalis cervicis; ijv, internal jugular vein; Isp, infraspinatus; L, labrum; LCo, longus colli; Lev, levator scapulae; LsC, longissimus cervicis; M, multifidus; MS, medulla spinalis; n, vagal nerve; RMj, rhomboid major; RMn, rhomboid minor; SA, subclavian artery; ScA, scalenus anterior; Scm, sternocleidomastoid; ScM, scalenus medius; ScP, scalenus posterior; SeC, semispinalis cervicis; SeCa, semispinalis capitis; Sh, sternohyoid; SpC, splenius cervicis; SpCa, splenius capitis; SrA, serratus anterior; SrP, serratus posterior; Ssp, supraspinatus; Tr, trapezius; va, vertebral artery.

muscle inserts on the first rib between the scalene tubercle and the groove for the subclavian artery.[42] It is the largest and longest scalene muscle. Its fascicle length ranges between 4.0 cm and 6.3 cm and its CSA is 2 cm^2.[32]

- There are no data regarding the IZs and functional compartmentalization of the scalenus medius muscle. Therefore, the authors recommend that BoTX injection should be performed at 1 point at the level of C6-C7 vertebrae (see **Fig. 3**).

Scalenus Posterior

- Scalenus posterior attaches to the posterior tubercles of the transverse processes of C4-C6 vertebrae. Inferiorly, the muscle inserts on the second rib.[42] Although it is known as the smallest of the scalene muscles, Kamibayasi and Richmond[32] found that the fascicle length changed between 4.5 cm to 6.5 cm and that the CSA of the scalenus posterior muscle was 1.55 cm^2.
- There are no data regarding the IZs and functional compartmentalization of the scalenus posterior muscle; therefore, the authors recommend that BoTX injection should be performed at 1 point at the level of T1 vertebra (see **Fig. 3**).

POSTERIOR NECK
Trapezius

- Trapezius muscle is anatomically subdivided into 3 parts: upper, transverse, and lower. Among them, the superior part and upper portion of the transverse part act on the cervical spine/head when the scapula is fixed. Although the upper part originates from superior nuchal line/ligament and attaches to the lateral third of the clavicula, the upper portion of the transverse part originates from C7 vertebra and inserts on the inner part of the acromion. The fascicles from the nuchal line down to C7 vertebra course inferiorly progressively with less steep orientation, such that fibers run almost horizontally at C7 vertebra.[42]
- Volumes and CSAs of the subdivisions of the upper part are 5 mL, 0.3 cm^2; 7 mL, 0.7 cm^2; 19 mL, 2.3 cm^2; and 20 mL, 2,2 cm^2 for the fascicles from the superior nuchal line, upper half of nuchal ligament, lower half of the nuchal ligament, and C6 and C7, respectively. The strongest fascicles of trapezius arise from C6 and C7 vertebrae. Length of the fascicles are 8 cm to 15 cm, 8 cm to 14 cm, 6 cm to 10 cm, and 6 cm to 11 cm for the superior nuchal line, upper half of the nuchal ligament, lower half of the nuchal ligament, and C7 vertebra, respectively.[32,42,43]
- Four functional compartments of the trapezius (uppermost, upper, uppermost lower, and lower) were detected using superficial EMG. Accordingly, the uppermost compartment originating from the nuchal line and nuchal ligament, and inserting on the clavicula corresponds to the anatomic upper part. The upper compartment aligned between the C7 vertebra and the acromion corresponds to the upper portion of the anatomic transverse part. It has been found that functional compartments are under independent voluntary control.[44] This means that all 4 compartments have distinct neuronal pools selectively innervating the related portion of the muscle. Therefore, in CD patients, dystonic involvement of the uppermost and upper functional compartments contributing to the head and neck movements may show significant differences. This is important in the clinical evaluation of CD patients and for the selection of muscle portions to apply BoTX injection.
- The IZs of trapezius muscle were found distributed in a narrow band lying along the midpoint of the muscle fibers.[45–47] As such, the authors recommend that BoTX injection to the trapezius muscle should be performed at 3 points at the middle of the muscle fascicles. Recommended points for uppermost, upper, and upper portions of the transverse parts are the midportions of the lines between C3 and one-third lateral portion of the clavicula, C6 and one-third lateral portion of the clavicula, and C7 vertebra and the acromion angle, respectively **(Fig. 4)**.

Levator Scapulae

- Levator scapulae attaches to the transverse processes of atlas and axis and the posterior tubercle of the transverse processes of the C3-C4 vertebrae. It descends inferolaterally with an angle of 30° to 45° to the midline and inserts on the medial border of the scapula.[32,42]
- Length of the fascicles ranges between 4.5 cm and 13.37 cm and its CSA is 2.18 cm^2.[32]
- No data about the IZs and functional compartmentalization of the levator scapulae exist; therefore, the authors recommend that BoTX injection should be performed at 1 point at the level of C6-C7 vertebrae.
  - Tatu and Jost[48] suggested that the muscle bundles originating from different transverse processes can be injected selectively (under US guidance) to act on the related vertebral level (see **Figs. 3** and **4**).

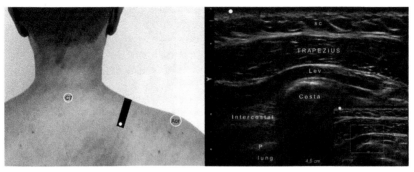

Fig. 4. When the probe is positioned in the sagittal (oblique) plane at midline between the C7 spinous process and the acromion, trapezius muscle is seen. Transverse cervical artery can also be visualized with power Doppler imaging (*inset*). Acr, acromion; Lev, levator scapulae; P, pleura; sc, subcutaneous tissue.

Splenius Capitis and Splenius Cervicis

- Splenius capitis is a large flat muscle originating from the mastoid process and lateral third of the superior nuchal line. It has parallel fascicles running inferomedially toward the posterior cervical midline. Upper fibers insert on the lower half of the nuchal ligament. Lower fibers attach to the spinous processes of C7-T4 vertebrae.[32]
- Splenius cervicis arises from the transverse processes of the first 3 cervical vertebrae and inserts on the spinous processes of T3-T6 vertebrae. As its fibers pass inferomedially, they wrap around other posterior intrinsic neck muscles.[42]
- Fascicle lengths of splenius capitis and cervicis range between 7.0 cm to 10.7 cm and 6.5 cm to 11.5 cm, respectively.
  - Kamibayashi and Richmond[32] did not mention any intramuscular aponeuroses or tendinous inscription, assuming that muscle fascicles elongate between their origins and insertions without interruptions.
- The CSA of splenius muscles is 4.26 cm². In the literature, no data concerning the functional compartmentalization of splenius capitis and cervicis muscle exist.
- In a recent study using surface EMG, IZ of splenius capitis was detected between 38.7% and 60% of the distance between the mastoid process and the sternal notch.[28] The IZ of semisipinalis cervicis is not known.
- The authors' recommendation for splenius capitis injections is at 2 points at the level of C2 vertebra for the upper medial part and at C5 vertebra for the lower lateral part. Because splenius cervicis has similar fascicle length but is narrower than capitis, 1-point injection is recommended for it at the level of C6 vertebra (**Figs. 5 and 6**).

Semispinalis Capitis and Semispinalis Cervicis

- Semispinalis capitis is a complex muscle having internal tendons and tendinous inscriptions. It originates from the medial part of occipital region between the superior and inferior nuchal lines and ends as flat tendons inserting into the superior articular processes of C4-C7 vertebrae and the transverse processes of T1-T6 or T7 vertebrae. It has thick muscle bundles that can easily be palpated just lateral to the nuchal ligament in the suboccipital region. It has 2 anatomic compartments: medial and lateral. In the medial compartment, fascicles attach to 3 to 4 incomplete tendinous inscriptions, which lay

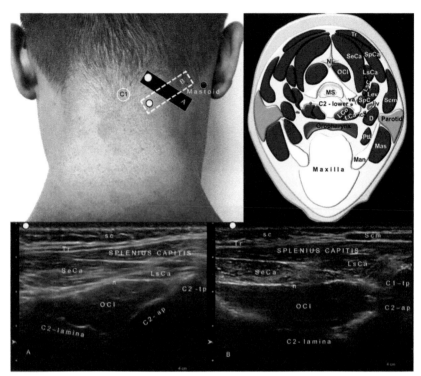

Fig. 5. When the probe is positioned in the axial (oblique) plane at C1-C2 level, splenius capitis and obliquus capitis inferior muscles can be seen (A). Greater occipital nerve can better be visualized at this level if the probe is shifted counter clockwise parallel to the long axis of obliquus capitis inferior (B). ap, articular process; D, digastric; ica, internal carotid artery; ijv, internal jugular vein; LCa, longus capitis; LCo, longus colli; Lev, levator scapulae; LsC, longissimus cervicis; LsCa, Longissimus capitis; Man, mandible; Mas, masseter; MS, medulla spinalis; n; greater occipital nerve; NL, nuchal ligament; OCI, obliquus capitis inferior; PtL, pterygoid lateralis; sc, subcutaneous tissue; SeCa, semispinalis capitis; Scm, sternocleidomastoid; SpC, splenius cervicis; SpCa, splenius capitis; tp, transverse process; Tr, trapezius; va, vertebral artery.

perpendicularly to fascicles at different levels in the upper half of the muscle. Some fascicles insert on the intramuscular aponeuroses. The medial compartment is formed by fascicles originating from thoracic vertebrae. Sometimes it is also called, biventer cervicis, assuming that there is only 1 inscription. The lateral compartment is semicircular in shape and although its fascicles course between the origin and insertions without any interruption, they have aponeuroses at the origin. Therefore, fascicle lengths in the 2 compartments are similar, 6.2 cm ± 1.1 cm.[32,48]

- Semispinalis cervicis originates from the spinous processes of C2-C5 vertebrae and, after spanning approximately 6 segments, inserts to the transverse processes of T1-T5 or T6 vertebrae.
- The literature lacks data concerning the IZs and functional compartmentalization of semispinalis capitis and cervicis muscles.
- The authors recommend that BoTX injections to semispinalis capitis should be performed at longitudinally arranged 2 points at the level of C1 and C3

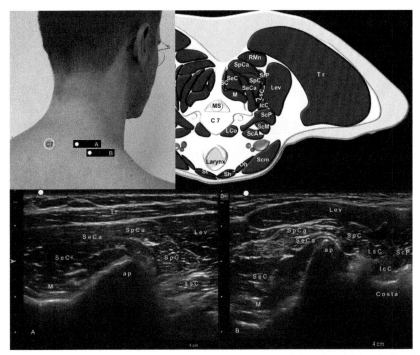

Fig. 6. When the probe is positioned in the axial plane at C7 (A) and T1 (B) levels, longissimus cervicis and iliocostalis cervicis muscles are seen. ap, articular process; Del, deltoid; IcC, iliocostalis cervicis; LCo, longus colli; Lev, levator scapulae; LsC, longissimus cervicis; M, multifidus; MS, medulla spinalis; Oh, omohyoid; RMn, rhomboid minor; SC, spinalis cervicis; ScA, scalenus anterior; Scm, sternocleidomastoid; ScM, scalenus medius; ScP, scalenus posterior; SeC, semispinalis cervicis; SeCa, semispinalis capitis; Sh, sternohyoid; SpC, splenius cervicis; SpCa, splenius capitis; SrP, serratus posterior; St, sternothyroid; Tr, trapezius.

vertebrae for the medial compartment (having tendinous inscriptions) and at 1 point at the level of C3 vertebra for the lateral compartment (having continuous fibers).

- The BoTX injection to semispinalis cervicis should be performed at 2 points at the level of C4 and C6 vertebrae (see **Fig. 5**; **Fig. 7**).

Longissimus Capitis

- Longissimus capitis is a narrow and flat muscle originating from the posterior aspect of the mastoid process. Its tendons insert on the transverse processes of C4-T4 vertebrae. Its musculotendinous length is between 13 cm and 18 cm.[32]
- There are no data about its IZs and compartmentalization; therefore, the authors recommend that BoTX injection to longissimus capitis should be performed at 2 points, at the levels of C1 and C3 vertebrae (**Fig. 8**).

Longissimus Cervicis and Iliocostalis Cervicis

- Longissimus cervicis originates from the posterior tubercles of the transverse processes of C2-C6 vertebrae and inserts on T1-T4 or T5 vertebrae. It is a long and thin muscle.

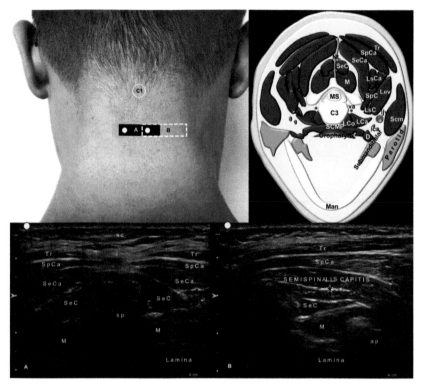

Fig. 7. When the probe is positioned in the axial plane at C3 level, semispinalis capitis muscle can be seen (A and B). The inscription of the muscle (*star*) can also/nicely be distinguished (B). ap, articular process; D, digastric; ica, internal carotid artery; ijv, internal jugular vein; LCo, longus colli; LCa, longus capitis; Lev, levator scapulae; LsCa, longissimus capitis; LsC, logissimus cervicis; M, multifidus, Man, mandible; MS, medulla spinalis; NL, nuchal ligament; sc, subcutaneous tissue; Scm, sternocleidomastoid; SCMP, superior constrictor muscle of pharynx; SeC, semispinalis cervicis; SeCa, semispinalis capitis; sp, spinous process; SpC, splenius cervicis; SpCa, splenius capitis; Tr, trapezius; va, vertebral artery.

- Iliocostalis cervicis originates from C4-6 vertebrae, descending over the posterior surface of the ribs, and attaches to the third to sixth ribs.[42]
- IZs and compartmentalization of these muscles are not known so the authors recommend that BoTX injection for these muscles should be performed at 1 point at the level of C7 for longissimus cervicis and at the level of T1 for iliocostalis cervicis (see **Fig. 6**).

Rectus Capitis Posterior Major and Rectus Capitis Posterior Minor

- Rectus capitis posterior major originates from the spinous process of axis and inserts on the lateral part of the inferior nuchal line and the occipital bone. As it ascends superolaterally, it becomes broader.
- Rectus capitis posterior minor originates from the tubercle on the posterior arch of the atlas and inserts on the medial part of the inferior nuchal line and the occipital bone. As it ascends, it becomes broader before its attachment. Either muscle may be doubled longitudinally.[42]

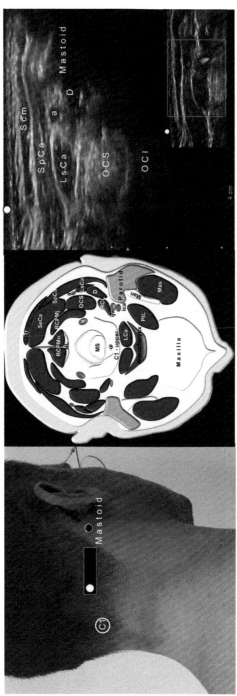

Fig. 8. When the probe is positioned in the axial plane medial to the inferior margin of the mastoid process, longissimus capitis and obliquus capitis superior muscles can be seen at C1-upper level. Occipital artery is nicely visualized in B-mode and power Doppler (*inset*) images. a, occipital artery; ica, internal carotid artery; D, digastric; ijv, internal jugular vein; LCa, longus capitis; LsCa, longissimus capitis; Mas, masseter; Man, mandible; MS, medulla spinalis; NL, nuchal ligament; o, odontoid process; OCI, obliquus capitis inferior; OCS, obliquus capitis superior; PtL, pterygoid lateralis; RCL, rectus capitis lateralis; RCPMj, rectus capitis posterior major; RCPMn, rectus capitis posterior minor; Scm, sternocleidomastoid; SeCa, semispinalis capitis; SpC, splenius cervicis; SpCa, splenius capitis; Tr, trapezius; v, vein.

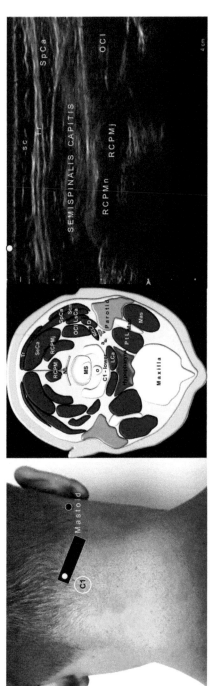

Fig. 9. When the probe is positioned in the axial (oblique) plane at occiput-C2 level, semispinalis capitis, rectus capitis posterior minor - major muscles can be seen. a, artery; D, digastric; Lev, levator scapulae; LCa, longus capitis; LsCa, longissimus capitis; Mas, masseter; Man, mandible; MS, medulla spinalis; NL, nuchal ligament; OCI, obliquus capitis inferior; OCS, obliquus capitis superior; PtL, pterygoid lateralis; RCL, rectus capitis lateralis; RCPMj, rectus capitis posterior major; RCPMn, rectus capitis posterior minor; sc, subcutaneous tissue; Scm, sternocleidomastoid; SeCa, semispinalis capitis; SpCa, splenius capitis; Tr, trapezius; v, vein.

Table 2
Commonly involved neck muscles in cervical dystonia and the suggested botulinum toxin injection sites

Neck Region	Muscle	Origin / Insertion	Adjacent Structures	N	Injection Level
Anterior	SCM	Manubrium (sternal head) and medial 1/3 of the clavicle (clavicular head) / Mastoid process, superior nuchal line	CCA, IJV, vagal nerve, spinal accessory nerve	4	30% 60% (from the mastoid process to the most medial point of the clavicle)
	Longus capitis	Transverse processes of C3-C6 / Basilar part of the occipital bone	CCA, IJV, vagal nerve, phrenic nerve, esophagus, thyroid gland, cervical sympathetic ganglion (superior (C2-3), middle (C6-7), inferior (C7-T1)), recurrent laryngeal nerve, nerve root, inferior thyroidal artery	1	C3
	Longus colli	Transverse processes of C3-T3 / Anterior arch of C1		2	C3 C6
Lateral	Scalenius anterior	Anterior tubercles of C3-C6 / 1st costa	Phrenic nerve, brachial plexus, EJV, subclavian artery, thyrocervical trunk and its branches	1	a C7/T1
	Scalenius medius	Posterior tubercles of C2-C7 / 1st costa		1	a C6/C7
	Scalenius posterior	Posterior tubercles of C4-C6 / 2nd costa	Spinal accessory nerve, branches of the cervical plexus	1	a T1
Posterior	Trapezius	External occipital protuberance, nuchal ligament, spinous processes of C1-T12	Spinal accessory nerve, branches of the cervical plexus, TON	3	Midportions of the 3 reference lines C3—lateral 1/3 of the clavicle C5—lateral 1/3 of the clavicle C7—acromion angle
	Levator scapulae	Transverse processes of C1-C4 / Medial border of the scapula	Lung apex, spinal accessory nerve	1	a C6/C7
	Splenius capitis	Nuchal ligament, spinous processes of C7-T4, and C7 vertebrae / Mastoid process, superior nuchal line		2	Medial portion at C2 Lateral portion at C5
	Splenius cervicis	Transverse processes of C1-C3		1	C6

(continued on next page)

Table 2
(continued)

Neck Region	Muscle	Origin / Insertion	Adjacent Structures	N	Level
	Semispinalis capitis	Spinous process of T3-T6; Transverse process of C7-T6 / The area between the superior and inferior nuchal lines	GON, TON	3	Medial portion at C1; Medial portion at C3; Lateral portion at C3
	Semispinalis cervicis	Transverse processes of T1-T6 / Spinous processes of C2-C5		2	C4; C6
	Longissimus capitis	Transverse processes of C4-T4 / Mastoid process	Occipital artery	2	C1; C3
	Longissimus cervicis	Transverse processes of C2-C6 / T1-T5 vertebrae		1	C7
	Iliocostalis cervicis	C4-6 vertebrae / 3rd to 6th costae		1	T1
	RCPMj	Spinous process of C2 / Inferior nuchal line	Vertebral artery, GON	1	[a]Occiput-C2
	RCPMn	Posterior tubercle of C1 / Inferior nuchal line		1	[a]Occiput-C1
	OCI	Spinous process of C2 / Transverse process of C1	Vertebral artery/vein, GON, TON, communicating cervical nerves	1	[a]C1-C2
	OCS	Transverse process of C1 / Lateral impression on the occiput	Vertebral artery, occipital artery	1	[a]Occiput-C1

Abbreviations: CCA, common carotid artery; EJV, external jugular vein; GON, greater occipital nerve; IJV, internal jugulary vein; N, number; OCI, obliquus capitis inferior; OCS, obliquus capitis superior; RCPMj, rectus capitis posterior major; RCPMn, rectus capitis posterior minor muscle; TON, third occipital nerve.
[a] The bulkiest site detected using US.

- The ranges of fascicle lengths are 2.0 cm to 4.1 cm and 1.5 cm to 2.0 cm, and PCSAs are 0.93 cm^2 and 0.50 cm^2 for rectus capitis posterior major and minor, respectively.[32] Both muscles have simple structures and their fascicles course in a slightly superolateral direction with an angle of 5°.
- The authors recommend that BoTX injection to rectus capitis posterior muscles should be performed at 1 point, that is, at the middle portion of the muscle belly at the level between C2 vertebra to occiput for major and C1 vertebra to occiput for minor (**Fig. 9**).

Obliquus Capitis Inferior and Obliquus Capitis Superior

- Obliquus capitis inferior originates from the spinous process and the lamina of the axis and inserts on the transverse process of atlas. It runs laterally and slightly cranial.
- Obliquus capitis superior originates from the transverse process of atlas and inserts on the occipital bone between the superior and inferior nuchal lines, overlapping the attachment of rectus capitis posterior major. It has 2 anatomic compartments. Although fascicles in the superficial compartment run along much of the muscle length, deeper fascicles are shorter and originate from an internal tendon.
- The ranges of fascicle lengths are 3.1 cm to 4.6 cm and 1.2 cm to 3.8 cm, and PCSAs are 1.29 cm^2 and 1.03 cm^2 for obliquus capitis inferior and superior, respectively.[32]
- The authors recommend that BoTX injections to oblique capitis muscles should be performed at single points, that is, at the midportion of the muscle belly at the level between C1 vertebra and occiput for oblique capitis superior (see **Fig. 8**) and between C2-C1 vertebrae for inferior (see **Fig. 5**).

All the commonly involved neck muscles in CD and the suggested BoTX injection sites are given in **Table 2**.

REFERENCES

1. Zoons E, Dijkgraaf MG, Dijk JM, et al. Botulinum toxin as treatment for focal dystonia: a systematic review of the pharmaco-therapeutic and pharmaco-economic value. J Neurol 2012;259:2519–26.
2. Albanese A, Abbruzzese G, Dressler D, et al. Practical guidance for CD management involving treatment of botulinum toxin: a consensus statement. J Neurol 2015;262:2201–13.
3. Bledsoe IO, Comella CL. Botulinum toxin treatment of cervical dystonia. Semin Neurol 2016;36:47–53.
4. Allison SK, Odderson IR. Ultrasound and electromyography guidance for injection of the longus colli with botulinum toxin for the treatment of cervical dystonia. Ultrasound Q 2016;32:302–6.
5. Jinnah HA, Goodmann E, Rosen AR, et al. Botulinum toxin treatment failures in cervical dystonia: causes, management, and outcomes. J Neurol 2016;263: 1188–94.
6. Lim EC, Seet RC. Botulinum toxin: description of injection techniques and examination of controversies surrounding toxin diffusion. Acta Neurol Scand 2008;117:73–84.
7. Costa J, Espírito-Santo C, Borges A, et al. Botulinum toxin type A therapy for cervical dystonia. Cochrane Database Syst Rev 2005;(1):CD003633.
8. Racette BA, Lopate G, Good L, et al. Ptosis as a remote effect of therapeutic botulinum toxin B injection. Neurology 2002;59:1445–7.

9. Hong JS, Sathe GG, Niyonkuru C, et al. Elimination of dysphagia using ultrasound guidance for botulinum toxin injections in cervical dystonia. Muscle Nerve 2012;46:535–9.
10. Dressler D. Electromyographic evaluation of cervical dystonia for planning of botulinum toxin therapy. Eur J Neurol 2000;7:713–8.
11. Nijmeijer SW, Koelman JH, Kamphuis DJ, et al. Muscle selection for treatment of cervical dystonia with botulinum toxin-a systematic review. Parkinsonism Relat Disord 2012;18:731–6.
12. Schramm A, Bäumer T, Fietzek U, et al. Relevance of sonography for botulinum toxin treatment of cervical dystonia: an expert statement. J Neural Transm (Vienna) 2015;122:1457–63.
13. Ross MH, Charness ME, Sudarsky L, et al. Treatment of occupational cramp with botulinum toxin: diffusion of toxin to adjacent noninjected muscles. Muscle Nerve 1997;20:593–8.
14. Comella CL, Jankovic J, Brin MF. Use of botulinum toxin type A in the treatment of cervical dystonia. Neurology 2000;55:S15–21.
15. Harry WG, Bennett JD, Guha SC. Scalene muscles and the brachial plexus: anatomical variations and their clinical significance. Clin Anat 1997;10:250–2.
16. Mayoux-Benhamou MA, Revel M, Wybier M, et al. Computerized tomographical study of dorsal neck muscles for insertion of EMG wire electrodes. J Electromyogr Kinesiol 1995;5:101–7.
17. Bhidayasiri R. Treatment of complex cervical dystonia with botulinum toxin: Involvement of deep-cervical muscles may contribute to suboptimal responses. Parkinsonism Relat Disord 2011;17(Suppl 1):S20–4.
18. Emsley JG, Davis MD. Partial unilateral absence of the trapezius muscle in a human cadaver. Clin Anat 2001;14:383–6.
19. Glass GA, Ku S, Ostrem JL, et al. Fluoroscopic, EMG-guided injection of botulinum toxin into the longus colli for the treatment of anterocollis. Parkinsonism Relat Disord 2009;15:610–3.
20. Özçakar L, Kara M, Chang KV, et al. Nineteen reasons why physiatrists should do musculoskeletal ultrasound: EURO-MUSCULUS/USPRM recommendations. Am J Phys Med Rehabil 2015;94:e45–9.
21. Chang KV, Şahin Onat Ş, Lee CW, et al. EURO-MUSCULUS/USPRM basic scanning protocols revisited in children. Eur J Phys Rehabil Med 2016;52:887–901.
22. Özçakar L, Kara M, Chang KV, et al. EURO-MUSCULUS/USPRM basic scanning protocols for hip. Eur J Phys Rehabil Med 2015;51:635–40.
23. Özçakar L, Kara M, Chang KV, et al. EURO-MUSCULUS/USPRM basic scanning protocols for ankle and foot. Eur J Phys Rehabil Med 2015;51:647–53.
24. Özçakar L, Kara M, Chang KV, et al. EURO-MUSCULUS/USPRM basic scanning protocols for knee. Eur J Phys Rehabil Med 2015;51:641–6.
25. Özçakar L, Kara M, Chang KV, et al. EURO-MUSCULUS/USPRM basic scanning protocols for wrist and hand. Eur J Phys Rehabil Med 2015;51:479–84.
26. Özçakar L, Kara M, Chang KV, et al. EURO-MUSCULUS/USPRM basic scanning protocols for elbow. Eur J Phys Rehabil Med 2015;51:485–9.
27. Özçakar L, Kara M, Chang KV, et al. EURO-MUSCULUS/USPRM basic scanning protocols for shoulder. Eur J Phys Rehabil Med 2015;51:491–6.
28. Delnooz CC, Veugen LC, Pasman JW, et al. The clinical utility of botulinum toxin injections targeted at the motor endplate zone in cervical dystonia. Eur J Neurol 2014;21:1486–98.
29. Kaymak B, Kara M, Yağız-On A, et al. Innervation zone targeted botulinum toxin injections. Eur J Phys Rehabil Med 2017. [Epub ahead of print].

30. Kaymak B, Kara M, Tok F, et al. Sonographic guide for botulinum toxin injections of the lower limb: Euro-musculus/USPRM spasticity approach. Eur J Phys Rehabil Med 2017. [Epub ahead of print].
31. Kara M, Kaymak B, Ulaşli AM, et al. Sonographic guide for botulinum toxin injections of the upper limb: Euro-musculus/USPRM spasticity approach. Eur J Phys Rehabil Med 2017. [Epub ahead of print].
32. Kamibayashi LK, Richmond FJ. Morphometry of human neck muscles. Spine (Phila Pa 1976) 1998;23:1314–23.
33. Paul AC. Muscle length affects the architecture and pattern of innervation differently in leg muscles of mouse, guinea pig, and rabbit compared to those of human and monkey muscles. Anat Rec 2001;262:301–9.
34. Elwischger K, Kasprian G, Weber M, et al. Intramuscular distribution of botulinum toxin-visualized by MRI. J Neurol Sci 2014;344:76–9.
35. Kennedy E, Albert M, Nicholson H. The fascicular anatomy and peak force capabilities of the sternocleidomastoid muscle. Surg Radiol Anat 2017;39(6):629–45.
36. Kim SY, Jang HB, Kim J, et al. Bilateral four heads of the sternocleidomastoid muscle. Surg Radiol Anat 2015;37:871–3.
37. Saha A, Mandal S, Chakraborty S, et al. Morphological study of the attachment of sternocleidomastoid muscle. Singapore Med J 2014;55:45–7.
38. McLoon LK. Muscle fiber type compartmentalization and expression of an immature myosin isoform in the sternocleidomastoid muscle of rabbits and primates. J Neurol Sci 1998;156:3–11.
39. Weeks OI, English AW. Compartmentalization of the cat lateral gastrocnemius motor nucleus. J Comp Neurol 1985;235:255–67.
40. Lee JH, Lee BN, Han SH, et al. The effective zone of botulinum toxin A injections in the sternocleidomastoid muscle. Surg Radiol Anat 2011;33:185–90.
41. Falla D, Dall'Alba P, Rainoldi A, et al. Location of innervation zones of sternocleidomastoid and scalene muscles-a basis for clinical and research electromyography applications. Clin Neurophysiol 2002;113:57–63.
42. Newell RLM. The back. In: Standring S, editor. Gray's anatomy. 40th edition. London: Elsevier; 2008. p. 707–73.
43. Johnson G, Bogduk N, Nowitzke A, et al. Anatomy and actions of the trapezius muscle. Clin Biomech (Bristol, Avon) 1994;9:44–50.
44. Holtermann A, Roeleveld K, Mork PJ, et al. Selective activation of neuromuscular compartments within the human trapezius muscle. J Electromyogr Kinesiol 2009;19:896–902.
45. Shiraishi M, Masuda T, Sadoyama T, et al. Innervation zones in the back muscles investigated by multichannel surface EMG. J Electromyogr Kinesiol 1995;5:161–7.
46. Xie P, Qin B, Yang F, et al. Lidocaine injection in the intramuscular innervation zone can effectively treat chronic neck pain caused by MTrPs in the trapezius muscle. Pain Physician 2015;18:E815–26.
47. Barbero M, Cescon C, Tettamanti A, et al. Myofascial trigger points and innervation zone locations in upper trapezius muscles. BMC Musculoskelet Disord 2013;14:179.
48. Tatu L, Jost WH. Anatomy and cervical dystonia: "Dysfunction follows form". J Neural Transm (Vienna) 2017;124:237–43.

Prolotherapy for the Thoracolumbar Myofascial System

Bradley D. Fullerton, MD[a,b,]*

KEYWORDS

- Prolotherapy • Thoracolumbar fascia • Interspinous ligament • PRP • Ultrasound
- Low back pain • Biotensegrity

KEY POINTS

- Prolotherapy has focused on entheses as a key source of chronic low back pain, even without clear diagnosis of enthesopathy.
- Treatment has traditionally been guided by anatomic knowledge and careful palpation. Dynamic ultrasonography can visualize tissue pathology previously identified only by detailed palpation.
- Prolotherapy cannot be fully understood without knowledge of biotensegrity and fascial anatomy.
- Biotensegrity provides the framework for a fundamentally different understanding of biomechanics, musculoskeletal diagnosis, and treatment.
- Detailed case studies of chronic pain resolution can provide proof of concept evidence for prolotherapy in the treatment of low back pain.

 Video content accompanies this article at http://www.pmr.theclinics.com.

PROLOTHERAPY: WHAT IS IT?

In the 1958 edition of his classic book on prolotherapy, Hackett described the treatment as a strengthening of "the weld of disabled ligaments and tendons to bone by stimulating the production of new bone and fibrous tissue cells..."[1] The 1939 research of Kellgren,[2] showing sciatic-like referral from the interspinous ligaments of the lumbar spine (**Fig. 1**), led Hackett to focus on ligaments as a source of pain

Disclosure Statement: The author has nothing to disclose.
[a] Private Practice: ProloAustin, 2714 Bee Cave Road, Suite 106, Austin, TX 78746, USA;
[b] Department of Internal Medicine, Texas A&M College of Medicine, Health Professions Education Building, 8447 Riverside Parkway, Bryan, TX 77807, USA
* Private Practice: ProloAustin, 2714 Bee Cave Road, Suite 106, Austin, TX 78746.
E-mail address: drbdf@aol.com

Phys Med Rehabil Clin N Am 29 (2018) 125–138
https://doi.org/10.1016/j.pmr.2017.08.010
1047-9651/18/© 2017 Elsevier Inc. All rights reserved.

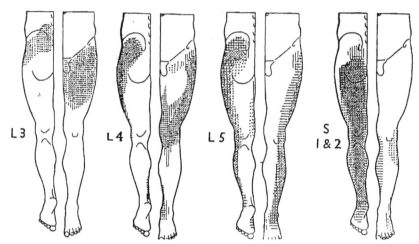

Fig. 1. A composite image adapted from Kellgren's original article showing referral patterns induced by injecting 0.1 mL to 0.3 mL of 6% saline into the interspinous ligament. At each level, the left image is a posterior view, whereas the right image is an anterior view. (*From* Kellgren JH. On the distribution of pain arising from deep somatic structures with charts of segmental pain areas. Clin Sci 1939;4(35):38; with permission.)

referral. He reasoned that stimulating repair in these structures could resolve long-standing low back and sciatic pain. He also performed his own experiments documenting the referral patterns of sacroiliac ligaments into the lower extremities (**Fig. 2**).[3]

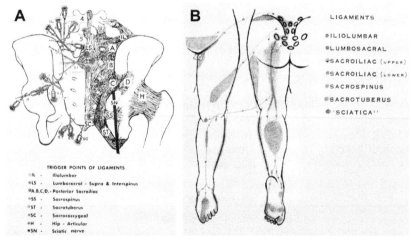

Fig. 2. A composite image of Hackett's original color diagrams documenting pain referral patterns with hypertonic saline injection into various ligaments supporting the sacroiliac joint. (*A*) indicates injection location whereas (*B*) indicates the referral patterns of those injections. (*From* Hackett GS, Hemwall GA, Montgomery GA. Ligament and tendon relaxation treated by prolotherapy. 5th edition. Madison (WI): Hackett Hemwall Patterson Foundation; 1993. p. 26–36. Available at: http://hhpfoundation.org/; with permission.)

As a result, the practice of prolotherapy has developed as a process of widespread injection of enthesis points using pain and crepitus to palpation as a guide to diagnosis and injection location. Yet, many of the anatomic structures injected have no known documented pathology and thus are not included in standard differential diagnosis. This has made study design difficult and opened the technique to significant criticism. The narrow focus on the disk as the most common cause of back pain continues to this day even in regenerative medicine circles.[4] If Kellgren and Hackett were correct, however, there are many tissues of the spine that are still minimized as potential sources of pain and, more importantly, as sources of abnormal biomechanics, which could contribute to degenerative spine conditions.

In 1995, *SPINE: State of the Art Reviews* published a volume on prolotherapy in the lumbar spine and pelvis. In that volume, Mooney, an orthopedic spine surgeon and one of the founding editors of the journal *Spine*, reported on his own experience of "the bias in the scientific community against innovative concepts" such as prolotherapy.[5] He touched on the difficulty of diagnosis in orthopedic medicine versus orthopedic surgery. He stated, "in contrast to fractures, each problem is somewhat different as to the location of the weak link." He encouraged readers to be open to new words and concepts such as "tensegrity … and particularly the integrated fascial system."

FASCIAL ANATOMY AND BIOTENSEGRITY

In the more than 20 years since that publication, this integrated fascial system have received extensive attention from fields, such as osteopathy and manual therapy/bodywork. In 2007, the first Fascia Research Congress met as an effort to bring together connective tissue research scientists and a diverse community of body workers.[6] In 2012, Willard and colleagues[7] published a thorough examination of the anatomy and function of the thoracolumbar fascia (TLF), which included a transverse section of the layers and sublayers of this structure. This image (**Fig. 3**) facilitates understanding of ultrasound images as discussed later in the case studies. This standardization of nomenclature for the TLF also reveals how this system integrates input from epaxial (spine), hypaxial (abdomen), and appendicular (the 4 extremities) myofascial systems. In 2015, Stecco[8] authored the first anatomic text focused on the continuity of the myofascial system throughout the body; she advocates for a slightly different nomenclature of the TLF.

The underlying biomechanics of this integrated fascial system have been explored by Stephen Levin, an orthopedic surgeon and systems scientist.[9] Levin expanded on concepts from futurist and architect Buckminster Fuller, who proposed the term, *tensegrity* (a combination of tension and integrity), to describe a class of constructs known as *floating compression* by the sculptor Kenneth Snelson (Video 1).

To understand structural stability with minimal mass, Fuller explained that "tension is primary and comprehensive, and compression is secondary and local."[10] Levin argues that traditional biomechanics, which involve lever forces and ultimately shear, will never fully explain the intrinsic mobility with stability of biologic structures. Levin proposed the term, *biotensegrity*, as the application of these concepts to biologic structures. In biotensegrity structures, there are no bending moments and no shear forces; thus, they have the lowest energy costs.

In the same volume of *SPINE: State of the Art Reviews*,[11] Levin stated that the sacrum and all other bones should be considered as compression-bearing structures, which float in a continuous network of tension supplied by fascia, muscles, ligaments, and other connective tissue. Thus, the soft tissues are the primary frame of the body, whereas the bones are islands within that continuous frame.

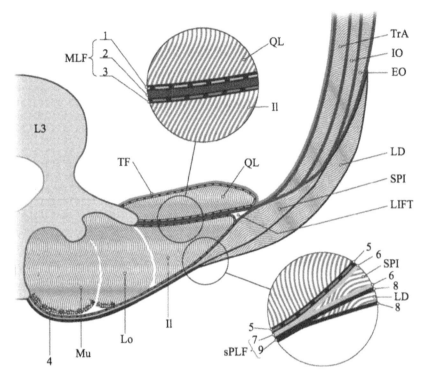

Fig. 3. Transverse view of TLF layers: This diagram correlates with an axial view of the traditional lumbar MRI. The patient is supine and the view is from caudal to cephalad of the left side. Willard and colleagues state, "This is a transverse section of the PLF and MLF and related muscles at the L3 level. Fascial structures are represented such that individual layers are visible, but not necessarily presented to scale." The details of each sublayer are beyond the scope of this review. Structures identified in the 2 case reports include hypaxial myofascia (the transversus abdominis [TrA] muscle and quadratus lumborum [QL]), epaxial myofascia (the 3 paraspinal muscles, multifidus [Mu], longissimus [Lo], and iliocostalis [II], which are deep to the PLF; all provide input into the aponeurosis of the erector spinae muscles [Apo ES] indicated as #4 and by a stippling pattern), and appendicular myofascia (latissimus dorsi [LD], serratus posterior inferior [SPI], and lower trapezius, which is not depicted at this level). The MLF is a combination of the hypaxial and epaxial myofascia. These layers are magnified in the upper circle of the diagram. The PLF is a combination of the epaxial and appendicular myofascia. These layers are magnified in the lower circle of the diagram. The LIFT is a combination of all 3 myofascial layers. The lateral raphe (not labeled) connects the abdominal wall muscles to the TLF; it includes the LIFT and tendon of the TrA. sPLF is superficial layer of PLF. IO is internal oblique. EO is external oblique. (*Adapted from* Willard FH, Vleeming A, Schuenke MD, et al. The thoracolumbar fascia: anatomy, function and clinical considerations. J Anat 2012;221(6):517; with permission.)

Biotensegrity structures are also fully integrated so that forces are instantaneously transferred through the entire structure. If the tension in the structure is continuous, any force applied to the structure deforms the entire structure. The structure itself then becomes a far more rapid form of communication than nerve conduction. When there is a loss of tension somewhere in the system, this communication is interrupted resulting in abnormal muscle recruitment and altered mobility. The task for the prolotherapist then becomes finding the loss of tensional integrity in the soft tissue frame and stimulating repair at the loss of tensegrity.

BIOTENSEGRITY-BASED ANATOMY AND BIOMECHANICS—A SUMMARY

1. Muscles are not structures that pull on bones to cause movement.
2. Bones float in a variable tension network consisting of muscle and fascial elements.
3. Fascial continuity provides passive tension and stored energy in the form of prestress.
4. Muscle fibers within the fascial continuity provide dynamic tension.
5. Thus, bones move (or, in the setting of outside forces, remained stable) when the tension around them changes.

CLINICAL APPLICATION OF BIOTENSEGRITY PRINCIPLES—A SUMMARY

1. Construct—focus on tensional continuity, which provides instantaneous, body-wide communication
2. History—past trauma is a loss of prestress in the tensegrity system
3. Signs/symptoms—muscle hyperactivity is compensation for loss of prestress (or loss of tensional continuity)
4. Diagnosis—use dynamics (in physical examination and ultrasonography) to find a loss of tensional continuity in the myofascia
5. Regenerative treatment—applied at the loss of tensional continuity (which may or may not be the location of a pain generator)

DETAILED CASE REPORTS AS PROOF OF CONCEPT

The complexity of biotensegrity structures and the complexity of prolotherapy treatments make large well-designed studies difficult. A recent review found only 2 studies of prolotherapy in low back pain that met criteria for inclusion.[12] With the large number of connective tissue structures as possible sources of pain and instability, even agreement on diagnosis among experienced practitioners can be difficult. These difficulties should not deter examining the decades of positive clinical reports concerning prolotherapy. It may be that the underlying pathology treated by prolotherapy would be better understood by detailed study of individual patients rather than starting with large controlled studies.

Case 1—Chronic Back Spasm Related to Injury of the Posterior Layer of the Thoracolumbar Fascia/Aponeurosis of the Erector Spinae Muscles/Interspinous Ligament/Multifidi Tendon

A 48-year-old white man with a greater than 10-year history of waxing and waning, activity-dependent low back pain and spasm without gluteal or lower extremity referral. Approximately 15 years prior to presentation he had an episode of his back locking up when flexed. He did not seek treatment and was able to recover over several days' time. These symptoms resolved and he was able to complete an iron man triathlon in the years after that. The onset of his chronic symptoms was gradual and initially seemed minor. Eventually he saw a chiropractor and had adjustments that did not affect his back pain. He sought consultation with an orthopedic spine surgeon; a lumbar MRI showed degenerative disk disease in the lower lumbar spine. These records were unavailable for review. In the year prior to his recurring back spasm, he was playing table tennis and felt a "pull" in his low back. Since that time, he has had daily low back pain, and exercise has been limited by recurring left lumbar muscle spasm. He is unable to complete lumbar strengthening exercises or participate in aerobic activities due to these back spasms.

Physical examination is remarkable for visually prominent left thoracolumbar paraspinals during single-leg stance. He is unsteady with single-leg squat bilaterally. In bipedal standing, there is a palpable deviation of the upper lumbar, posterior spinous processes toward the right. In supine position, he is unable to maintain straight leg raise (SLR) against resistance bilaterally. In prone position, there is palpable crepitus and tenderness on the left side of the upper lumbar spinous processes but none on the right. This correlated with ultrasound findings (Video 2). In prone he has difficulty but can partially maintain SLR against resistance bilaterally. With prone hip external rotation against resistance, he is unable to maintain stability at the midlumbar spine. His spine rotates at that location when testing either right or left. Otherwise, lower extremity strength, sensation, and muscle stretch reflexes are normal. There are no neural tension signs and lumbar range of motion is only mildly limited in flexion.

Ultrasound examination is focused at midline lumbar spine with linear-array high-frequency transducer. This revealed a cortical pit at the L1 posterior spinous process with thickening of the posterior layer of the TLF (PLF) on the left compared with the right (**Fig. 4**). With sonographic palpation (Video 3), the left longissimus lumborum

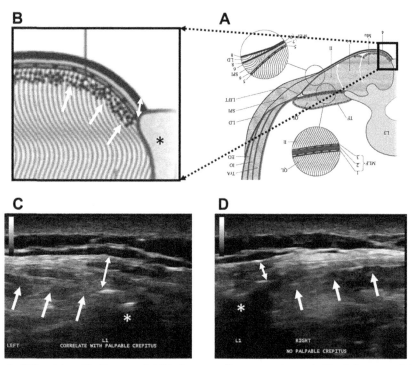

Fig. 4. PLF and Apo ES ultrasound. (*A*) is the same diagram as shown in **Fig. 3**; however, it has been reversed to correlate with the view seen on ultrasound when the patient is in the prone position. The view is still from caudad to cephalad viewing the left side. (*B*) Magnified view of the same diagram correlating with the black box in (*A*). (*C, D*) Ultrasound images of the patient in case 1. In *B, C* and *D*, single-head arrows point to the Apo ES, which is irregular and poorly defined on the left compared with the right. In *B, C* and *D*, double-head arrows indicate the thickness of the PLF at the insertion into the L1 posterior spinous process, with cortical pit indicated by (*asterisk*). The left PLF is thickened and heterogenous compared with the right. ([*A, B*] *Adapted from* Willard FH, Vleeming A, Schuenke MD, et al. The thoracolumbar fascia: anatomy, function and clinical considerations. J Anat 2012;221(6):517; with permission.)

fibers partially collapse and translate laterally. The right longissimus lumborum fibers maintain stability with compression and do not translate laterally (**Fig. 5**). At lower lumbar levels, the multifidi appeared partially torn at the spinous process and blending with the aponeurosis of the erector spinae muscles (Apo ES). This is seen most clearly with compression at L5 (Video 4).

Treatment involved initial injection of a solution of 0.3% lidocaine and 15% dextrose at the tissues of interest under ultrasound guidance, then repeat of physical examination maneuvers to evaluate response. This was then repeated for other structures until the patient was pain-free and had normal dynamic testing (**Box 1**). The same structures are then injected with a total of 4-mL low–white blood cell, low–red blood cell, autologous platelet-rich plasma (PRP) derived from 60 mL of whole blood.

At follow-up 2.5 months after procedure, the patient reported significant improvement in his chronic pain. He described having no back pain the day after the procedure and states, "that was really interesting." Then the pain returned to its normal baseline; 6 weeks to 8 weeks later, he noticed the episodes of activity-limiting pain and spasm were decreasing. In discussing the back pain, he reported, "I always feel it" but "it doesn't get in my way now." He has been able to run up to 2 miles without increase in back pain and estimates overall improvement at 50%.

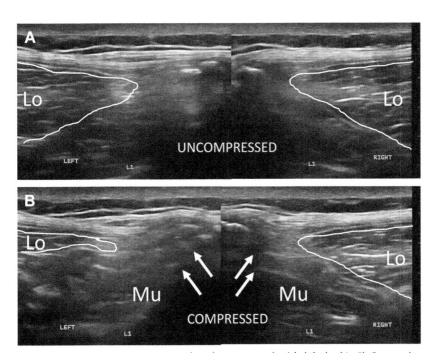

Fig. 5. Longissimus at L1 uncompressed and compressed with labels. (*A*, *B*) Composites of still images taken from Video 3 with the posterior spinous process at the midline. Longissimus (Lo) is outlined in white. At upper lumbar levels the longissimus fibers extend more medially overlying the multifidus (Mu). In (*A*), the uncompressed left side is farther from the spinous process than the uncompressed right. In (*B*), the left longissimus compresses easily and translates farther lateral compared with the right. The arrows point toward the blending of multifidus tendon into the Apo ES, which are also more heterogenous and hypoechoic on the left compared with the right.

Box 1
Case 1, structures injected

1. Left PLF and Apo ES at L1 and L2 spinous processes (Video 5)
2. L1-2 and L2-3 supraspinous and interspinous ligaments (Video 6)[13]
   a. After injection of 1 and 2, supine and prone SLR strength against resistance was normal and without pain
   b. Prone hip external rotation strength testing showed improved control of lumbar rotation.
3. Left multifidus insertions at L3-5 posterior spinous processes (Video 7)
   a. After injection 3, prone hip external rotation strength testing showed complete stability of lumbar rotation.

On examination, there is no palpable deviation of the upper lumbar, posterior spinous processes toward the right in bipedal standing. There is no tenderness to palpation and minimal crepitus in this area. He had full strength with prone SLR against resistance. There was still mild lumbar rotation with prone hip external rotation against resistance. Ultrasonography showed clear improvements in tissue organization and resistance to sonographic compression (Video 8). The plan was to continue increasing activity to tolerance and follow-up in 2 months if pain returned or progress plateaued.

He did not return for follow-up. At phone follow-up 2.5 years' posttreatment, he reported that the pain and spasm had continued to reduce over the several months after the last appointment. He has had no back spasms, even with increased activity, over the past 2.5 years. He says he is approximately 75% better compared with before treatment and has no limitations from his back pain.

Case 1 discussion
Prolotherapy in the lumbosacral spine is a purposefully broad injection pattern that seems imprecise to those unfamiliar with the technique. In the lumbar spine, common injection locations include the posterior and lateral surfaces of the posterior spinous processes, the lateral and posterior surfaces of the transverse processes, facet joint capsules, iliolumbar ligament insertions at the ilium, and sacroiliac ligaments indicated on the Hackett diagram (see **Fig. 2**). A similar standardized injection pattern was used in a randomized controlled study by Yelland and colleagues.[14] The conclusion of this article states, "in chronic nonspecific low back pain, significant and sustained reductions in pain and disability occur with ligament injections, irrespective of the solution injected or the concurrent use of exercises." Although this study was performed more than 12 years ago, ligament injection to treat chronic nonspecific low back pain is offered by few physicians. Understanding ligament and other connective tissue pathology may motivate more physicians to learn this method.

The approach described in this case is a hybrid of traditional prolotherapy injection location (informed by history and physical examination findings) with ultrasound diagnosis and ultrasound guidance to clarify the pathology traditionally treated with prolotherapy. The laxity in the Apo ES and the overlying PLF could have resulted from the acute episode of the pull while playing table tennis and/or the chronic, repetitive trauma of his exercise regimen with breakdown of collagen fibers. Using tensegrity theory, the recurring muscle spasms in this patient are interpreted as an attempt by the body to reintroduce prestress into these fascial layers. The laxity in these collagen layers would conceivably change the length-tension relationship of the muscles that insert into these layers. This would alter the timing of muscle recruitment and cause repetitive abnormal stresses to other tissues, such as the disks, over time.

In the author's experience, prolotherapy to the interspinous ligament (as in this case) can result in remarkable clinical improvements. The misunderstood anatomy of the interspinous ligaments may provide some explanation for this observation. Classic anatomy texts[15,16] describe the interspinous ligaments as connecting adjacent posterior spinous processes. As described by Willard,[13] however, the interspinous ligament fibers are in parallel with the spinous processes; thus, they connect the supraspinous ligament to the ligamentum flavum. The fanlike fibers are narrow as they blend with the ligamentum flavum and become broader as they blend with the supraspinous ligament. During lumbar flexion, this arrangement transmits tension from the TLF/supraspinous ligament to the ligamentum flavum, resulting in elevation of the ligamentum flavum away from the spinal canal (**Fig. 6**). Because the ligamentum flavum also blends with the facet capsules, the interspinous ligament transmits tension to those capsules as well. This may have profound implications in the understanding of ligamentum flavum buckling on MRI and the development of degenerative lumbar stenosis.

If injection of dextrose and PRP stimulates formation of collagen and return of prestress to the system, the muscle spasms should gradually reduce in the months after treatment as in this case. If the tissue diagnosis and injection location or correct, the clinical results should be long lasting, as in this case and the study by Yelland and colleagues[14]

Case 2—Recurring Sciatica Versus Pseudosciatica from Injury to Lumbar Interfascial Triangle and Gluteus Minimus/Medius

A 52-year-old woman with a 5-month history of right low back and gluteal pain referring to posterior lateral thigh and calf. This started after performing a headstand in

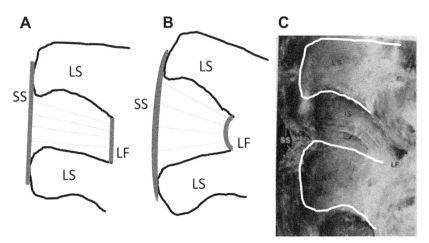

Fig. 6. Interspinous ligament anatomy and biomechanics. (C) A gross anatomy picture from Willard; the original image has been adapted by outlining the lumbar posterior spinous processes (LS) in white. (A) Shows the spine in neutral; (B) shows the spine in flexion. The thick lines correspond to the supraspinous ligament (SS) and ligamentum flavum (LF); the thin lines represent the fan shaped pattern of the interspinous ligament (IS) fibers. Note that in flexion, the IS fibers serve to transmit tension from SS to LF resulting in elevation of the LF away from the spinal canal. ([C] *Adapted from* Willard F. The muscular, ligamentous and neural structure of the lumbosacrum and its relationship to low back pain. In: Vleeming A, Mooney V, Dorman T, et al, editors. Movement, stability and low back pain: the essential role of the pelvis. New York: Churchill Livingstone; 1997. p. 7; with permission.)

yoga while pulling the legs up over her head; 2 months prior to this office visit, she had been diagnosed by a board-certified physiatrist with right lumbosacral radiculopathy; MRI indicated "Right paracentral disk herniation at L5-S1 inferior extrusion contacting the right S1 nerve root, Schmorl's node at the inferior aspect of the L5 vertebral body." She was given a "prednisone taper" and referred for lumbar extension–based therapy, which had been partially effective.

She also recalled 2 prior injuries. Six years previously, when learning to wakeboard, she was resisting being pulled up into a standing position when she felt a "pop" in her right low back and immediate pain and collapsed into lumbar and hip flexion. She had to be carried from the shore line to her car and required evaluation in an emergency room. She received an unknown injection and recovered over several days. Five years previously, she flipped over the handlebars of her mountain bike landing on the right low back causing significant abrasion and permanent scar near the posterior superior iliac spine.

At my initial evaluation, she continued to have sciatic pain (**Fig. 7**A) with an equivocal right SLR, absent right Achilles reflex, and normal strength and sensation. She was referred for physical therapy with focus on core strengthening and progressed well yet without resolution. She managed her chronic low back/hip pain using a lumbar pillow when sitting and remained active, including extended hiking vacations over the next 15 months. At that time, she had recurrence of the severe symptoms with sciatic referral (**Fig. 7**B) after performing a yoga strengthening exercise involving supine position, 90° hip flexion, and then maximal lumbar rotation side to side. She initially sought evaluation with the previous physician, who found recurrence of the positive SLR and recommended epidural steroid injection or evaluation for surgery on the herniated disk.

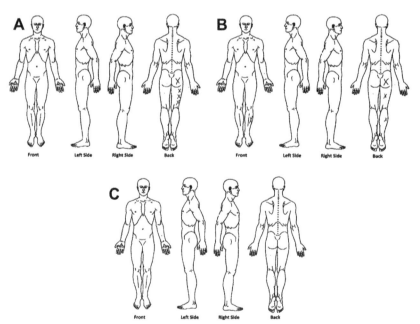

Fig. 7. Sequential pain diagrams of patient presenting with diagnosis of radiculopathy. (*A*) At the initial evaluation. Pain improved with physical therapy and she returned more than 1 year later with severe exacerbation. (*B*) At the time of representation and treatment with dextrose/PRP prolotherapy. (*C*) At 3-month follow-up posttreatment.

She sought a second opinion at my office, where physical examination was remarkable for standing posture with mild hip flexion; limited active lumbar range of motion in flexion, extension and left lateral flexion; unstable right single-leg squat; weak hip abduction and extension; positive right SLR at 35°; and tenderness to palpation at the right quadratus lumborum, right lateral gluteal muscles/ilium, and right gluteus medius tendon at the posterior facet of the greater trochanter. Sensation and lower extremity muscle stretch reflexes were normal.

Ultrasonography of the TLF system revealed a loss of tensional integrity in the right longissimus lumborum, quadratus lumborum, middle layer of the TLF (MLF) (**Fig. 8**, Video 9), lumbar interfascial triangle (LIFT), and lateral raphe at L4 (**Fig. 9**, Video 10). Ultrasonography of the right gluteal muscles revealed a loss of tensional integrity in the proximal musculotendinous junction of the gluteus medius, origin of the posterior part of the gluteus minimus from the ilium, and an intrasubstance partial tear of the gluteus medius tendon at the posterior facet of the greater trochanter.

Treatment involved initial injection of a solution of 0.3% lidocaine and 15% dextrose at the tissues of interest under ultrasound guidance and then repeat of dynamic physical examination maneuvers to evaluate response. This was then repeated for other structures until the patient was pain-free and had normal testing (**Box 2**). The same structures are then injected with a total of 10-mL low–white blood cell, low–red blood cell, autologous PRP derived from 120 mL of whole blood.

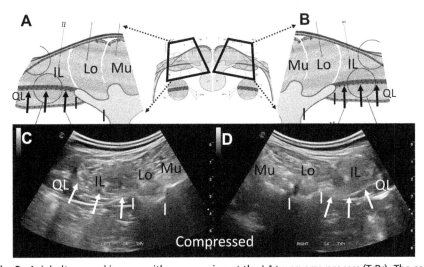

Fig. 8. Axial ultrasound images with compression at the L4 transverse process (TrPr). The center of (*A*, *B*) is a composite image using the transverse view of the TLF from Willard and colleagues, showing left and right sides of a prone patient. The lateral parts of (*A*) and (*B*) are a magnified image corresponding to the black trapezoids at the center, as indicated by the black dotted arrows. The trapezoids represent the section visualized on the curved-array ultrasound images in (*C*, *D*) (*left* and *right*, respectively). The length of the L4 TrPr is demarcated by the vertical white lines in the lower images and vertical black lines in the upper images. The MLF attaches to the tip of the TrPr (a common location of injection in prolotherapy); it is indicated by the white arrows in the lower images and the black arrows in the upper images. Note the poor definition of the compressed MLF and quadratus lumborum (QL) on the right compared with the left. Other muscles identified in *A–D* include multifidus (Mu), longissimus (Lo) and iliocostalis (IL). See Video 9 showing compression at this location. ([*A, B*] *Adapted from* Willard FH, Vleeming A, Schuenke MD, et al. The thoracolumbar fascia: anatomy, function and clinical considerations. J Anat 2012;221(6):517; with permission.)

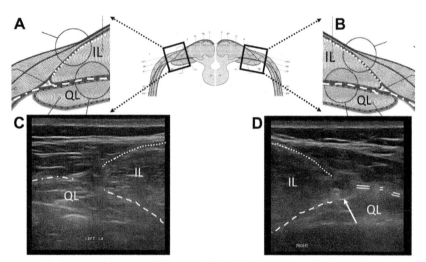

Fig. 9. Axial ultrasound images of bilateral LIFT at L4. The center of (*A*) and (*B*) is a composite image as in **Fig. 8**. The lateral parts of (*A*) and (*B*) are a magnified view corresponding to the black squares at the center, as indicated by the dotted arrows. The black squares represent the linear-array ultrasound images in (*C*) and (*D*) (*left* and *right*, respectively). The dotted white lines correspond to the PLF. The dashed white lines corresponding to the MLF. The dot–dash white lines correspond to the tendon of transversus abdominus (note the *right side* in [*D*] is a *wider line* indicating the poor definition compared with the *left* in [*C*]). These lines terminate at the 3 apices of the LIFT, which is also poorly defined on the right compared with the left. The white arrow points to the part of the LIFT that appears partially torn in Video 10, a video of compression in these locations. IL, iliocostalis muscle.

Over the next month, she experienced gradual reduction in sciatic pain and increase in walking tolerance. By 6 weeks' posttreatment, her sciatica was resolved and she had no pain with sitting or driving. At 3-month follow-up, she reported that she no longer thought about using her lumbar pillow during sitting and that she was pain-free with all activities (**Fig. 7**C). Right single-leg squat, SLR, and hip abduction/extension strength were all normal.

Box 2
Case 2, structures injected

1. Right lateral raphe from abdominal wall to LIFT and MLF at L4-5 (Video 11)
   a. After numbing here, supine SLR improved from 35° to 45° hip flexion with less radicular pain. Patient also reported decreased pain with lumbar flexion and increased stability with right single-leg squat.
2. Right gluteus medius musculotendinous junction
3. Right posterior part of the gluteus minimus origin at the ilium
   a. After numbing structures 2 and 3, there was no change in hip abduction strength. SLR was still positive at 45° hip flexion.
4. Right gluteus medius tendon at lateral and posterior facets of the greater trochanter
   a. After numbing structure 4, hip abduction strength was 5/5 and supine SLR was negative to 90°.

Case 2 discussion
Typical examination prior to palpation-guided prolotherapy includes a detailed palpation of the sacroiliac ligaments and the enthesis of all gluteal muscles, including the iliac crest, posterior superior iliac spine, lateral sacrum, lateral ilium, and greater trochanter. If tenderness is found, injection is performed at these locations as well. Most experienced prolotherapists have resolved cases of chronic low back pain with and without sciatica by treatment of mainly hip structures. What tissue pathology is being treated in these cases?

It is well known that trigger points in gluteus medius and minimus muscles can refer to the low back, lateral thigh, lateral leg, and foot.[17] During traditional prolotherapy technique, the gluteus medius and minimus are needled extensively when injecting the lateral ilium origins. The tendons are also routinely injected at the greater trochanter. The development of ultrasonography has allowed diagnosis and injection within myofascial structures that do not include attachment to bone, such as the LIFT and gluteus medius musculotendinous junction in this case.

This case illustrates the need to address multiple structures to resolve chronic referred pain, like the concept of a double-crush injury to the nerve. The diagnosis of radiculopathy was not necessarily incorrect. The forces that created the disk herniation and potential dynamic impact to the nerve root could have resulted from the multiple soft tissue injuries she sustained prior to the development of the radiculopathy. Once both injuries were addressed, the dynamics affecting the nerve root may have changed enough for her to become asymptomatic.

SUMMARY/FUTURE DIRECTIONS

Biological structures diffuse forces in ways that are not fully understood by biomechanical theory. Biotensegrity theory argues that forces are distributed to all the tissues of the body regardless of the trauma. If accurate, this seems to open all collagen fibers of the body to the level of potential diagnoses after trauma. Increasing knowledge of fascial anatomy is advancing understanding of previously ignored connections, such as the myofascial expansions described by Stecco.[8] Thus, the limitation of tissue diagnosis to small regions within the spine, such as the disk or facets, inevitably miss some of the loss of tension caused by trauma. Refinement of diagnosis as described in these cases will allow physicians to commonly diagnose injuries to soft tissue structures, such as LIFT, PLF, Apo ES, MLF, and the seemingly endless other soft tissue structures of the spine. More thorough understanding of how forces are transferred through these tissues in normal motion and in trauma will allow more rapid diagnosis of structures currently considered unimportant. Then, it may be possible to identify common patterns of myofascial injury and degeneration that predate commonly diagnosed degenerative conditions of the spine and extremities, such as disk degeneration and facet arthropathy.

SUPPLEMENTARY DATA

Supplementary data related to this article can be found online at https://doi.org/10.1016/j.pmr.2017.08.010.

REFERENCES

1. Hackett GS. Ligament and tendon relaxation treated by prolotherapy. 3rd edition. Springfield (IL): Charles C Thomas; 1958.

2. Kellgren JH. On the distribution of pain arising from deep somatic structures with charts of segmental pain areas. Clin Sci 1939;4:35–46.
3. Hackett GS, Hemwall GA, Montgomery GA. Ligament and tendon relaxation treated by prolotherapy. 5th edition. Madison (WI): Hackett Hemwall Patterson Foundation; 1993. p. 26–36. Available at: http://hhpfoundation.org/.
4. Mascarinas A, Harrison J, Boachie-Adjei K, et al. Regenerative treatments for spinal conditions. Phys Med Rehabil Clin N Am 2016;27(4):1003–17.
5. Mooney V. Prolotherapy in the spine and pelvis: an introduction. SPINE: State of the Art Reviews 1995;9(2):309–11.
6. Findley T, Schleip R. "Fascia research." Basic science and implication for conventional and complementary health care. Munich (Germany): Elsevier Health Sciences; 2007.
7. Willard FH, Vleeming A, Schuenke MD, et al. The thoracolumbar fascia: anatomy, function and clinical considerations. J Anat 2012;221(6):507–36.
8. Stecco C. Functional atlas of the human fascial system. London: Churchill Livingstone; 2015. p. 199–212.
9. Scarr G. Biotensegrity: the structural basis of life. Pencaitland (Scotland): Handspring Publishing; 2014.
10. Fuller B. Synergetics. New York: Macmillian; 1975.
11. Levin S. The sacrum in three-dimensional space. SPINE: State of the Art Reviews 1995;9(2):381–8.
12. Reeves KD, Sit RWS, Rabago DP. Dextrose prolotherapy: a narrative review of basic science, clinical research, and best treatment recommendations. Phys Med Rehabil Clin N Am 2016;27(4):783–823.
13. Willard F. The muscular, ligamentous and neural structure of the lumbosacrum and its relationship to low back pain. In: Vleeming A, Mooney V, Dorman T, et al, editors. Movement, stability and low back pain: the essential role of the pelvis. New York: Churchill Livingstone; 1997. p. 7–8.
14. Yelland MJ, Glasziou PP, Bogduk N, et al. Prolotherapy injections, saline injections, and exercises for chronic low-back pain: a randomized trial. Spine 2004; 29:9–16.
15. Spalteholz W. Hand-atlas of human anatomy. 7th edition in English. Philadelphia: Lippincott; 1943. p. 176.
16. Grant JCB. An atlas of anatomy. Baltimore (MD): Williams and Wilkins; 1956. p. 363.
17. Travell J, Simons D. Myofascial Pain and Dysfunction: The Trigger Point Manual. Volume 2: The Lower Extremities. Baltimore (MD); 1992. p. 151, 169.

Radiofrequency Denervation of the Cervical and Lumbar Spine

 CrossMark

Jessica Arias Garau, MD*

KEYWORDS

- Radiofrequency • Facet • Cervical • Lumbar • Medial branch • Third occipital nerve

KEY POINTS

- Facet joint nerve blocks help in the diagnosis of facet-related pain and are used to determine if patients are candidates for radiofrequency denervation.
- Radiofrequency denervation is a treatment modality that produces an electric current to coagulate and interrupt nerve transmission.
- Radiofrequency denervation can provide significant improvement in cervical and lumbar facet joint pain.

Facet or zygapophysial joint pain is a common cause of chronic neck and back pain in the population.[1] The prevalence of chronic neck pain in adults is approximately 15%.[2] A systematic review by Meucci and colleagues[3] demonstrated that the prevalence of chronic low back pain increases with age, particularly after 30 years of age, and is commonly seen in women. Facet joint pain occurs as a result of aging and degeneration. Degeneration causes dehydration of the discs, which results in decreased disc height, increased vertebral mobility, and increased shear forces on the facet joints.[4,5] Facetogenic pain is typically provoked on extension of the spine and may present clinically with axial, nonradicular pain affecting the cervical, thoracic, or lumbosacral spine. In 1941, Badgley[5] suggested that the facet joints could be primary sources of pain, independent of pain produced by spinal nerve compression. Multiple mechanisms have been proposed to explain facetogenic pain. Among these are stretching of the capsule around the facet joint, release of inflammatory mediators, synovial villi entrapment between articular surfaces, and nerve impingement by osteophytes.[6]

Facet joint pain is tested by performing a series of diagnostic blocks, which consist of injecting or bathing the facet joint nerve (medial branches) with local anesthetic.

Disclosure Statement: The author has nothing to disclose.
Advanced Orthopedics and Sports Medicine Institute, Pond View Professional Park, 301 Professional View Drive, Building 300, Freehold, NJ 07728, USA
* 2 Chelsea Avenue, Apartment 202, Long Branch, NJ 07740.
E-mail address: sinq09@yahoo.com

Phys Med Rehabil Clin N Am 29 (2018) 139–154
https://doi.org/10.1016/j.pmr.2017.08.011   pmr.theclinics.com
1047-9651/18/© 2017 Elsevier Inc. All rights reserved.

A positive test increases the likelihood that the facet joints are a primary source of pain and might enable the selection of patients who might respond to radiofrequency neurotomy. A negative test will exclude them as pain generators.[5,7–9] Once the pain source has been determined, radiofrequency denervation or neurotomy can be performed.

Studies have shown that performing medial branch blocks is the most reliable and appropriate way to diagnose facet-related pain.[10] There is still controversy in regard to what is the standard diagnostic protocol to select patients for radiofrequency denervation. How many blocks should be performed and what is the ideal cutoff (in terms of numeric scale for percent relief) to label a block as positive are some of the questions that still need to be further established with more certainty. According to Holtz and Sehgal,[1] radiofrequency denervation showed improvement in pain and disability scores, but no correlation was found between the response to diagnostic medial branch blocks and pain relief after radiofrequency neurotomy. This study suggests that the criteria for the number of blocks needed in order to select patients for this modality of treatment is still unclear.

In general, patients receiving greater than 50% relief after a diagnostic block have a better outcome, in terms of pain relief, with radiofrequency ablation than those with less than 50%. Previous studies have shown no significant difference in terms of radiofrequency denervation outcomes between the 50% and 80% cutoff values. Local anesthetic blocks providing greater than 80% relief increase the number of true positives and screen out the false negatives and the patients who have multiple pain generators.[1,11–13] A systematic review by Manchikanti and colleagues[10] showed that the prevalence of the accuracy and reliability of diagnostic facet medial branch blocks in the low back was 27% to 41% with a false-positive rate of 25% to 44% and the prevalence for the cervical spine was 36% to 67% with a false-positive rate of 27% to 63%. The study also concluded that diagnosing facet joint pain with diagnostic blocks is reliable and that treatment with therapeutic techniques, such as medial branch blocks, intraarticular facet injections, and radiofrequency ablations, can provide a significant improvement in facet joint pain.[2,10]

EQUIPMENT

- Radiofrequency denervation consists of guiding an insulated needlelike cannula toward the bony landmarks of the target nerve, typically using fluoroscopy. This modality of treatment is thought to produce Wallerian degeneration of the afferent nerve fibers, causing interruption of the nerve's normal function.[14] Radiofrequency denervation has been used for many years in Europe and other countries. Although most studies have shown improvement of zygapophysial joint pain, more published studies are needed in order to better understand its efficacy in the spine.
- The radiofrequency denervation equipment consists of a generator that delivers an alternating current to the body through a dispersion pad (**Fig. 1**). It produces an electric current that alternates at the radiofrequency of radio waves to coagulate and interrupt nerve transmission. The distal tip of a specialized insulated cannula is placed parallel over the target nerve to produce a lesion at maximal length. The lesion is created in the form of an oblate spheroid, and it might extend up to 2 mm away from the active tip.[15,16] An electric field is produced, increasing the temperature of the surrounding tissues and resulting in denervation or Wallerian degeneration of myelinated and unmyelinated nerve fibers.[14] Radiofrequency neurotomy is thought to denature the chemical components of the Aδ

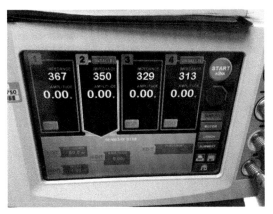

Fig. 1. Radiofrequency denervation generator.

and C nerve fibers preventing the pain signal conduction. Over time, the nerve recovers and regenerates in a proximal to distal direction. Pain may return, and repeated radiofrequency treatments may be performed.

- The duration of the radiofrequency denervation effect is related to the target nerve length and varies depending on the nerve diameter, course, neuro-anatomy, and the size of the lesions created.[17]
  ○ Increasing the exposed length of the metal active tip, the size of the needle, lesioning time, needle placement, and repeated lesioning can all increase the size of the lesion.[18]
  ○ The most commonly used cannula is the Sluijter (Radionics Inc. Burlington, MA)-Mehta cannula. It is usually a 22-gauge cannula and 5, 10, or 15 cm in length; it can cause lesions of 4, 5, or 10 mm.[4] For most patients, a 10-cm cannula must suffice.
  ○ A study by Cosman and colleagues[19] demonstrated that when the active tip is heated at 80°C for 90 seconds, a 23-gauge electrode with a 4-mm active tip produces lesions that average 5.9 mm long and 3.9 mm wide and a 16-gauge electrode with a 6-mm active tip produces a lesion that is 10.5 mm long and 9.2 mm wide. In this study, the 16-gauge electrode was the preferred electrode for cervical medial branch radiofrequency ablation.
- Other methods of radiofrequency denervation are used in pain management, such as pulsed and cooled radiofrequency. For the purpose of this article, the authors focus on conventional radiofrequency ablation.

CERVICAL FACET ANATOMY

- The zygapophysial (facet or z joints) are true diarthrodial synovial joints. They are composed of 2 opposing articular cartilaginous surfaces covered by a fibrous capsule enclosing the joint space. Facet joints are formed by the inferior articular process of the superior vertebrae and the superior articular process of the one below. These paired structures exist on each side of the cervical, thoracic, and lumbar spine to assist with segmental motion and weight bearing.[4,20]
- Anatomists have disagreed on the origins of certain structures innervating the cervical facets, but they have all concluded that facet joints are innervated and that they have the capability of producing pain.
- Histologically speaking, nerve-associated substances, such as substance P, and calcitonin gene-related peptide are thought to play a role in the pain pathway.[21]

The facet joint capsules contain mechanoreceptors and free nerve endings that are also thought to play an essential role in proprioception and pain sensation.[22]
- The anatomy and innervation for C1 to C2 is different from C3 to C8.
  - The atlas (C1) superior facets face downward and outward and articulate with the occipital condyles, whereas the inferior facets articulate with the superior facets on the axis.
  - The axis superior articular facets face upward and outward and articulate with the atlas.
  - The lower cervical facet joints (C3–C7) have a 45° angle orientation from the horizontal plane and an 85° angle from the sagittal plane, which prevent anterior translation and are important for weight bearing.[23]
  - The anterior and posterior rami innervate the cervical facet joints.
    - The C1 and C2 joints are innervated by the anterior rami of the first and second spinal nerves.
    - The C2-C3 facet is innervated by the communicating branch and the medial branch of the posterior ramus of the third spinal nerve or third occipital nerve (TON). Fibers from the TON also provide sensation to the suboccipital region.
    - The nerve supply for the lower cervical facets (C3–C4 to C7–T1) arises from the posterior rami medial branches from one level above and one level below for each individual facet joint.[24] The medial branches wrap around the waist of the articular pillars, which are the anatomic landmarks for facet medial branch blocks and radiofrequency denervation.

OCCIPITAL NEURALGIA AND CERVICOGENIC HEADACHE

- Chronic neck pain and occipital and cervicogenic neuralgias, including headaches, are commonly seen in the general population and in pain management practices. The prevalence of occipital neuralgia and cervicogenic headaches has been reported to range from 0.4% to as high as 16.0%.[25] It is important to properly identify and treat these conditions because if left untreated they might become refractory. Biondi and Bajwa,[26] Govind and colleagues,[27] and Hamer and Purath,[25] demonstrated that TON radiofrequency ablation is technically achievable and successful up to 5 to 6 months after treatment of patients with third occipital neuralgia.

INDICATIONS

- TON block and radiofrequency denervation can be used for the diagnosis and treatment of TON headaches. Patients with occipital neuralgia might complain of stabbing, lancinating, or sharp pain in the suboccipital region, often referred to the ipsilateral distribution of the V1 trigeminal nerve. The patients have associated spasms, neck pain, and tightness. Patients who have not responded to conservative treatment, including physical therapy, and have responded successfully to local anesthetic blocks of the TON are candidates for radiofrequency denervation.
- Some studies have shown controversy regarding this modality of treatment. A recent study by Wahezi and colleagues[28] mentioned that many patients with a cervicogenic headache who undergo radiofrequency neurotomies do not experience as much relief as they experienced with the diagnostic medial branch blocks. They investigated the underlying cause of the high number of false positives and found that the currently recommended injectate volumes (between 0.3

and 0.5 mL) used to block the TON might be blocking the greater occipital nerve (GON) as well. Therefore, performing radiofrequency denervation over the TON will only lesion a diameter of 5 to 7 mm and will not include the GON. They are suggesting consideration of radiofrequency lesioning over the TON and the GON for cervicogenic headache treatment. This study had some limitations, in particular the information translated from cadaveric findings to the clinical setting, its small sample size, and research bias.[28]

- Other studies, such as the one performed by Hamer and Purath,[25] demonstrated that radiofrequency denervation of the C2 dorsal root ganglion and/or TON can provide about 5 to 6 months of greater than 50% relief in most patients receiving the treatment.
- Despite the controversy, radiofrequency of the TON has been commonly performed and has been useful in the treatment of TON headaches.

TECHNIQUE: THIRD OCCIPITAL NERVE RADIOFREQUENCY DENERVATION

- Patients are placed in the prone position with the cervical spine in a slightly flexed position. A true lateral view with proper alignment of the C2-C3 articular pillars must be obtained. The overlying skin is prepped and draped in a sterile fashion, and local anesthetic is used to anesthetize the skin and subcutaneous tissues. A radiofrequency probe with a 22-gauge, 10-mm active tip, insulated blunt curved needle is inserted and directed under fluoroscopic visualization toward the midpoint between the opposite apex of the superior articular process of C3 and the opposite base of the C2-C3 neural foramen.
- Even though it is not strictly necessary if proper technique and careful fluoroscopic evaluation of the final needle position is obtained, motor and sensory stimulation should be performed for safety reasons to assure proper placement of the needle and avoid stimulating the nerve root. Motor stimulation is executed at 2 Hz with 0.5 to 1.5 V. There should be no motor stimulation of the ipsilateral facial or upper extremity. Sensory stimulation at 50 Hz with 0.1 to 0.75 V should elicit a paresthesia in the distribution of the TON. Negative aspiration of cerebrospinal fluid or blood must be obtained before injecting preservative-free local anesthetic. Patients must then be observed for at least 60 seconds before performing radiofrequency lesioning, to avoid intravascular or subarachnoid injection. Radiofrequency lesioning can then be executed for 90 seconds at 80°C.[29]

COMPLICATIONS

- Neuropathic pain might be a common complication after TON, C2-C3 radiofrequency denervation. A study by Gazelka and colleagues[30] reported an incidence of 19% neurotomy-induced occipital neuralgia in patients who presented with burning, tingling, or numbness after undergoing a TON or C2-C3 radiofrequency neurotomy. The anatomic proximity of the TON to the exiting spinal nerves places these structures at a high risk for puncture injury.
- Subarachnoid, subdural, or epidural injection and trauma might also occur.
  - Inadvertent injection through the foramen magnum into the subarachnoid space might result in total spinal anesthesia or even death.[17]
- Intravascular injection of local anesthetic may cause central nervous system side effects.[17]
- Other side effects may include numbness in a small area behind the ear that is supplied by the TON, temporary ataxia, dysesthesias, and itching.[17]

CERVICAL FACET RADIOFREQUENCY DENERVATION

- A systematic review by Engel and colleagues[17] reported that cervical radiofrequency neurotomy effectiveness is of high quality and that it has a low risk for complications. Most studies demonstrated almost complete pain relief at 6 months and up to 1 year in more than a third of the patients. The literature review also demonstrated that cervical radiofrequency denervation allows patients to return to work and to be able to perform previous activities that were limited by pain.[17,31]
- The target nerve for cervical radiofrequency neurotomy is the medial branch of the posterior dorsal rami. Patients who have responded favorably and receive pain relief to medial branch blocks for the duration of the local anesthetic are candidates for this procedure. Practitioners perform either single or double blocks. Others use different local anesthetics and compare the duration of the response with the duration of action of the local anesthetic.[7,8]
- The systematic review by Engel and colleagues[17] reports that obtaining positive results of comparative medial branch blocks is the only method that is validated for the diagnosis of facet joint pain.
- Clinically, patients with cervical facetogenic pain may complain of neck pain, headaches, or supraclavicular or shoulder pain (**Fig. 2**).

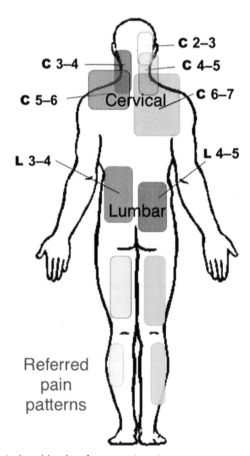

Fig. 2. Referred cervical and lumbar facetogenic pain patterns.

APPROACH

- When performing cervical medial branch blocks with local anesthetic, a posterior or lateral approach may be performed.
  - The lateral approach is more comfortable for patients in terms of positioning. Patients are placed in a lateral decubitus position with a pillow under the neck. The C-arm is placed in an anteroposterior (AP) view with perfect alignment of the left and right articular pillars. The C-arm remains in the same position throughout the procedure. The skin is anesthetized and advanced toward the midpoint of the articular pillar, and local anesthetic is injected to bathe the medial branch nerve. Some physicians prefer the lateral approach because the needle cuts through less amount of tissue to reach the target nerve. The disadvantage of this approach is the increased risk of driving the needle into the spinal canal, particularly if the bilateral facets are not lined up properly under the fluoroscope or if patients rotate the neck during the procedure.
  - Cervical medial branch radiofrequency denervation can also be performed using a posterior approach, which allows a better parallel alignment of the active tip along the target nerve on the articular pillar.[4,29,32] Patients are placed in the prone position for the posterior approach. A small headrest under the forehead and a chest pillow can be used to maximize patient comfort. The neck should be in a slightly flexed position. In order to better visualize the articular pillars, the C-arm should be tilted caudally until the axis of the x-rays is lined up with the facet joints. Counting the vertebrae, either from T1 upward or from C2 downward, is important in order properly identify the levels where the procedure will be performed. T1 is easily identified because of its large transverse processes and C2 because of the odontoid process. First, the skin and subcutaneous tissues are anesthetized with 1% lidocaine. Then, a radiofrequency cannula is inserted, directed, and advanced toward the articular pillar, coaxial to the x-ray beam. Once the radiofrequency cannula contacts the periosteum, the needle is walked off the facet and advanced 2 to 3 mm to properly place the cannula parallel to the medial branch (**Fig. 3**). In order to confirm the final placement of the needle, an AP, foraminal contralateral oblique and a lateral view may be obtained. In the AP view, the needle should be placed at the waist or lateral groove of the articular pillar. (see **Fig. 3**; **Fig. 4**). The foraminal contralateral oblique and the lateral views both must show the needle placement posterior to the neural foramen[32] (**Fig. 5**). Motor and sensory testing is also performed at all levels in order to confirm proper needle placement. The stimulation is carried out at 50 Hz, and patients should report pain or tingling during stimulation between 0.1 V and 0.5 V. No motor stimulation of the upper extremity should be seen at 2 Hz at no less than 2.5 to 3.0 times the sensory stimulation threshold. Motor stimulation of the affected myotome is an indicator that the needle might be in close proximity to the spinal nerve and must be repositioned. Each level is then anesthetized with preservative-free local anesthetic, and radiofrequency lesioning is performed at 80°C for 60 to 90 seconds (**Fig. 6**). The time of the denervation may vary among practitioners. Others might reposition the needle and perform multiple lesions at each level because of the anatomic variation of the medial branches to assure maximal therapeutic effect.[4,29]

COMPLICATIONS

- The systematic review presented by Engel and colleagues[17] listed the risks and complications following cervical radiofrequency ablation that were recorded in

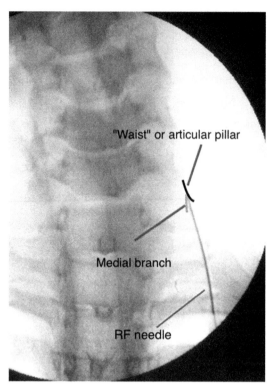

Fig. 3. AP view: cervical facet medial branch radiofrequency denervation. The radiofrequency cannula must be placed parallel to the medial branch for proper lesioning of the medial branch. RF, radiofrequency.

the literature and their prevalence with 95% confidence intervals. In order of frequency, complications included minimal radiation risks, temporary postprocedural pain, cutaneous numbness, dizziness, ataxia, dysesthesias, pruritus, postprocedural infection, vasovagal syncope, neuritis, and dermoid cysts. Some theoretic risks that have been discussed include radiation exposure, allergic reactions, bruising, ground electrode burns, neuroma, anesthesia dolorosa, and risks associated with implanted electrical devices.

LUMBAR FACET ANATOMY

- The lumbar facet joints are innervated by the dorsal rami of the lumbar spinal nerves L1 through L5.
  - A review article from Kozera and Ciszek[33] describes the division of the posterior branch into the medial and lateral branches about 5 to 10 mm distal to the opening bounded by the upper and lower edges of the adjacent transverse processes at an angle of 30°. The medial branch supplies innervation from the midline to the facet joint line, and the lateral branch supplies innervation to the surrounding tissues located lateral to the facet joint. An intermediate branch has also been described, and it supplies innervation to the longissimus muscle. The posterior branch of the L5 nerve differs from the aforementioned branches. It sends branches that cross the sacral ala between the lateral sacral

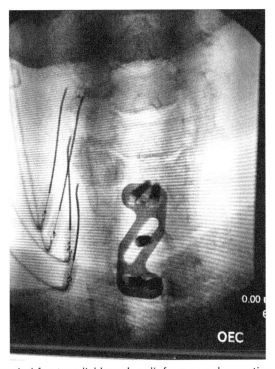

Fig. 4. AP view: cervical facet medial branch radiofrequency denervation.

bone and the medial superior area of the S1 superior articular process[33,34] (**Fig. 7**).

- Patients might complain of decreased extension and pressure or pain across the low back, hip, buttocks, and even referred pain in the posterior thighs (see **Fig. 2**).
- The medial branch of the dorsal ramus is targeted for block and denervation at the junction of the lateral aspect of the superior articulating process and the origin of the transverse process. The nerve enters a fibro-osseous canal bounded by the mammillary process, the accessory process, and the mamillo-accessory ligament.
  - According to Shuang and colleagues,[35] the medial branch is located closer to the medial aspect of the accessory process and farther from the lateral aspect of the mammillary process in the fibro-osseous canal.
- As mentioned earlier, in order to perform radiofrequency neurotomy of the L5 dorsal ramus, the needle must be directed toward the junction between the sacral ala and the superior articular process, parallel to the nerve.
- It is important to remember that when a block is performed for a facet joint, the medial branch of the same segment as well as the segment above need to be targeted in order to provide relief. Precise and accurate positioning of the needle for medial branch blocks and cannula for radiofrequency denervation is critical for successful treatment of facetogenic pain.

LUMBAR FACET RADIOFREQUENCY DENERVATION

- In patients who have been properly selected, lumbar radiofrequency denervation has shown great results in decreasing facet-related pain, improvement in quality

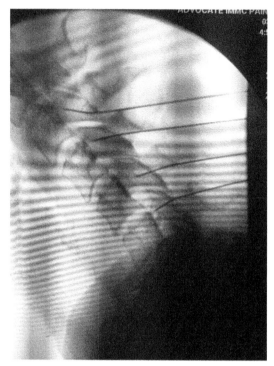

Fig. 5. Lateral view: cervical facet medial branch radiofrequency denervation.

of life, and reduction in analgesic doses.[35,36] Indications for radiofrequency lumbar facet denervation include patients with chronic low back pain that is refractory to conservative treatment but responsive to diagnostic medial branch blocks. Contraindications include ongoing infection or coagulopathies. Radiofrequency denervation may be performed in patients who have undergone spine

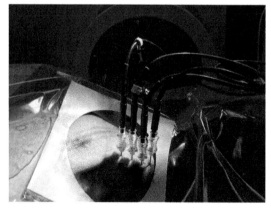

Fig. 6. Cervical facet radiofrequency lesioning is performed at 80°C for 60 to 90 seconds after proper testing is carried out and local anesthetic has been injected.

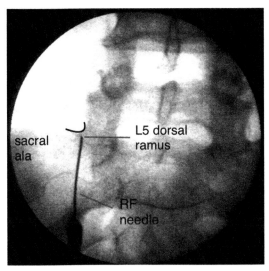

Fig. 7. The L5 dorsal ramus crosses the sacral ala between the lateral sacral bone and the medial superior area of the S1 superior articular process. RF, radiofrequency.

surgery, but scar tissue and hardware might prevent proper lesioning of the medial branch.[18]

TECHNIQUE

- Patients are positioned in the prone position, and a pillow may be placed under the abdomen to minimize the lumbar curvature and tilt the pelvis posteriorly.[4,29] First, the superior vertebral end plates are lined up. The lumbar level is then identified, by counting upward from the sacrum or downward from T12.
- The C-arm is then positioned at 15° to 30° of oblique angulation to better visualize the junction between the transverse process and the superior articulating process, which is the location for the medial branch.
- The skin and subcutaneous tissues are anesthetized with 1% lidocaine, and a radiofrequency cannula is guided under fluoroscopic visualization toward the junction between the superior articulating process and the transverse process of the level to be performed (**Fig. 8**). A caudal tilt may facilitate parallel positioning of the radiofrequency cannula over the medial branch. In the lateral view, the needle should be posterior to the neural foramen (**Fig. 9**).
- Once the radiofrequency cannula contacts the periosteum, the needle is walked off the facet and advanced 2 to 3 mm in order to properly place the cannula parallel to the medial branch. Following proper needle placement, motor and sensory stimulation is performed. Patients should feel stimulation, pressure, or discomfort at the low back, buttocks, or hips but not in the lower extremities.
  - This sensory stimulation must be decreased to less than 0.4 V at 5 Hz. Radicular pain or pattern experienced by patients is an indicator that the needle must be repositioned, because it might be in close proximity to the spinal nerve.
  - Motor stimulation at 2 Hz between 2.0 V and 2.5 V must produce contraction of the multifidus muscles in the back and no motor stimulation of the lower extremities. Again, if motor stimulation is seen in the lower extremities, the needle

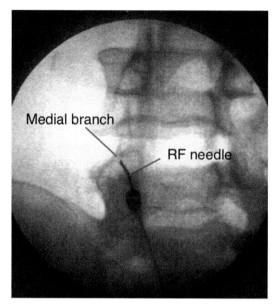

Fig. 8. Lumbar facet radiofrequency denervation. The active tip radiofrequency cannula should be placed between the superior articulating process and the transverse process of the level to be performed. RF, radiofrequency.

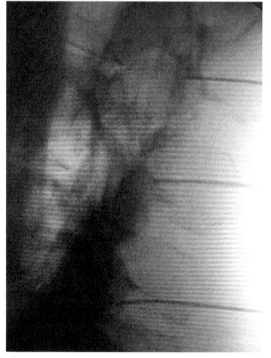

Fig. 9. Lateral view: lumbar medial branch radiofrequency denervation.

needs to be repositioned because of the close proximity of the needle to the spinal nerve.
- Once the testing is completed and the needle position is confirmed, local anesthetic is injected into each level and radiofrequency denervation is carried out at 80°C for 60 to 90 seconds (**Fig. 10**). Some physicians might perform multiple lesions after slight repositioning of the needle.

COMPLICATIONS

- According to Shuang and colleagues,[35] the distance between the dorsal ramus bifurcation and the superior border of the root of the transverse process is approximately 3 mm and the dorsal ramus is only 1 cm away from the ventral ramus. Therefore, when performing medial branch blocks or radiofrequency denervation, one should be careful not to advance the needle 3 mm superior to the root of the transverse process.
- Repeated puncture may result in nerve injury secondary to the proximity of the ventral ramus, permanent lower extremity weakness, neuritis, or permanent sensory deficits. Bleeding or hematoma may occur with accidental vessel puncture.
- Another complication that might occur is spinal instability and multifidus muscle denervation, if performed in excess. Therefore, radiofrequency should be limited to 3 or less spinal segments.[35]
- The literature shows that an increase in low back pain after the procedure may occur in about 1% of the patients.[37,38]

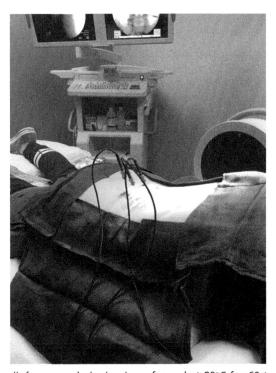

Fig. 10. Lumbar radiofrequency lesioning is performed at 80°C for 60 to 90 seconds after proper testing is carried out and local anesthetic has been injected.

TECHNICAL TIPS TO IMPROVE RADIOFREQUENCY DENERVATION

- Understanding the principles and technicalities of how radiofrequency works is essential for any interventional pain management physician. It is important to remember that radiofrequency denervation produces a coagulation effect over the target nerve by using a cannula that transmits an electric current. Proper alignment of the needle in a parallel fashion with the nerve is important to get maximal lesioning and better results. The physician must possess vast knowledge about the neuroanatomy of spine and the target nerves in order to be able to guide the needle with more accuracy toward the bony landmarks and avoid serious complications.
- The C-arm must be aligned properly for each level in order to better visualize the structures.
- The needle should be advanced coaxial to the x-ray beam, which will facilitate directing the needle toward the target area in a timely fashion. The coaxial approach minimizes the need for needle redirection which sometimes might increase post procedure discomfort.
- Make sure to choose the correct cannula with the appropriate lesion size for the spinal segment being treated.
- Some physicians might decrease the procedure time by using radiofrequency generators with multiple cannulas that can be launched at the same time after proper motor and sensory testing has been performed.
- Finally, it is of extreme importance to keep a sterile technique to avoid infections and other complications from the procedure.

SUMMARY

Analysis of the evidence by Manchikanti and colleagues[10] demonstrated that radiofrequency denervation was able to reduce pain by 50% in at least 50% of the patients with a relative risk of side effects and adverse events. The evidence is fickle in regard to radiofrequency denervation for the cervical and lumbar spine. The effectiveness for lumbar facet radiofrequency denervation is evidence level I for less than 6 months and level II for 6 months or longer. For the cervical spine, the evidence is level II.[10] Overall, radiofrequency neurotomy is a safe and effective technique used to treat facet-related pain. It is important to remember that controlled diagnostic medial branch blocks are essential to confirm that the facet joints are the primary pain generators before proceeding with radiofrequency denervation for longer-term treatment in patients with chronic axial low back pain.[4,18]

REFERENCES

1. Holtz SC, Sehgal N. What is the correlation between facet joint radiofrequency outcome and response to comparative medial branch blocks? Pain Physician 2016;19(3):163–72.
2. Falco FJ, Manchikanti L, Datta S, et al. Systematic review of the therapeutic effectiveness of facet joint interventions: an update. Pain Physician 2012;15(6): E839–68.
3. Meucci RD, Fassa AG, Xavier NM. Prevalence of chronic low back pain: systematic review. Rev Saude Publica 2015;49:1.
4. Rathmel JP. Atlas of image-guided intervention in regional anesthesia and pain medicine. Philadelphia: Lippincott Williams & Wilkins; 2006. p. 65–92.

5. Badgley CE. The articular facets in relation to low back pain and sciatic radiation. J Bone Joint Surg 1941;23:481.
6. Bykowski JL, Wong WH. Role of facet joints in spine pain and image-guided treatment: a review. AJNR AM J Neuroradiol 2012;33:1419–26.
7. Barnesley L, Lord S, Bogduck N. Comparative local anesthetic blocks in the diagnosis of cervical zygapophysial joint pain. Pain 1993;55:99–106.
8. Barnesley L, Lord S, Wallis B, et al. False-positive rate of cervical zygapophysial joint blocks. Clin J Pain 1993;9:124–30.
9. Kaplan M, Dreyfuss P, Halbrook B, et al. The ability of lumbar medial branch blocks to anesthetize the zygapophysial joint. A physiologic challenge. Spine (Phila Pa 1976) 1998;23:1847–52.
10. Manchikanti L, Kaye A, Boswell MV, et al. A systematic review and best evidence synthesis of effectiveness of therapeutic facet joint interventions in managing chronic spinal pain. Pain Physician 2015;18:E535–82.
11. Derby R, Melnik I, Lee JE, et al. Correlation of lumbar medial branch neurotomy results with diagnostic medial branch block cutoff values to optimize therapeutic outcome. Pain Med 2012;13:1533–46.
12. Cohen SP, Strassels SA, Kurihara C, et al. Establishing an optimal "cutoff" threshold for diagnostic lumbar facet blocks: a prospective correlational study. Clin J Pain 2013;29:382–91.
13. Cohen SP, Stojanovic MP, Crooks M, et al. Lumbar zygapophysial (facet) joint radiofrequency denervation success as a function of pain relief during diagnostic medial branch blocks: a multicenter analysis. Spine J 2008;8:498–504.
14. Smith HP, McWhorter JM, Challa VR. Radiofrequency neurolysis in a clinical model. Neuropathological correlation. J Neurosurg 1981;55:246–53.
15. Lau P, Mercer S, Govind J, et al. The surgical anatomy of lumbar medial branch neurotomy (facet degeneration). Pain Med 2004;5:289–98.
16. Schofferman J, Kine G. Effectiveness of repeated radiofrequency lumbar neurotomy for lumbar facet pain. Spine 2004;29:2471–3.
17. Engel A, Rappard G, King W, et al. The effectiveness and risks of fluoroscopically guided cervical medial branch thermal radiofrequency neurotomy: a systematic review with comprehensive analysis of the published data. Pain Med 2016; 17(4):658–69.
18. Mazin DA, Sullivan JP. Lumbar and sacral radiofrequency neurotomy [review]. Phys Med Rehabil Clin N Am 2010;21(4):843–50.
19. Cosman ER Jr, Dolensky JR, Hoffman RA. Factors that affect radiofrequency heat lesion size. Pain Med 2014;15:2020–36.
20. Windsor RE, Falco FJE. Clinical orientation to spinal anatomy. Atlanta (GA): O2 Communications Inc; 2003. p. 85–8.
21. Youseff P, Loukas M, Chapman JR, et al. Comprehensive anatomical and immunohistochemical review of the innervation of the human spine and joints with application to an improved understanding of back pain. Childs Nerv Syst 2016; 32(2):243–51.
22. McLain RF. Mechanoreceptor endings in human cervical facet joints. Spine 1994; 19(5):495–501.
23. Bland J. Disorders of the cervical spine. Philadelphia: WB Saunders Co; 1987.
24. Bogduk N. The clinical anatomy of the cervical dorsal rami. Spine 1982;7(4): 319–29.
25. Hamer J, Purath T. Response of cervicogenic headache and occipital neuralgia to radiofrequency ablation of the C2 dorsal root ganglion and/or third occipital nerve. Headache 2014;54:500–10.

26. Biondi D, Bajwa Z. Cervicogenic headaches. UpToDate.com: Wolters Kluwer Health; 2013.
27. Govind J, King W, Bailey B, et al. Radiofrequency neurotomy for the treatment of third occipital headache. J Neurol Neurosurg Psychiatry 2003;74:88–93.
28. Wahezi SE, Silva K, Shaparin N, et al. Currently recommended TON injectate volumes concomitantly block the GON: clinical implications for managing cervicogenic headache. Pain Physician 2016;19(7):E1079–86.
29. Waldman SD. Atlas of interventional pain management. Philadelphia: Elsevier Saunders; 2015. p. 157–77, 473–88.
30. Gazelka HM, Knievel S, Mauck WD, et al. Incidence of neuropathic pain after radiofrequency denervation of the third occipital nerve. J Pain Res 2014;7:195–8.
31. Basset K, Sibley LM, Anton H, et al. Percutaneous radiofrequency neurotomy treatment of chronic cervical pain following whiplash injury: reviewing evidence and needs. Vancouver: British Columbia Office of Health Technology Assessment; 2001. p. 40–7.
32. Furman MB, Lee TS, Berkwits L. Atlas of image-guided spinal procedures. Philadelphia: Elsevier Saunders; 2013. p. 141–8, 279–94.
33. Kozera K, Ciszek B. Posterior branches of lumbar spinal nerves-part I: anatomy and functional importance. Ortop Traumatol Rehabil 2016;18(1):1–10.
34. Bodguk N, Wilson AS, Tynan W. The human lumbar dorsal rami. J Anat 1982; 134(2):383–97.
35. Shuang F, Hou SX, Zhu JL, et al. Clinical anatomy and measurement of the medial branch of the spinal dorsal ramus. Medicine 2015;94(52):1–5.
36. Lakemeier S, Lind M, Schulz W, et al. A comparison of intra-articular lumbar facet joint steroid injections and lumbar facet joint radiofrequency denervation in the treatment of low back pain: a randomized, controlled, double-blind trial. Anesth Analg 2013;117:228–35.
37. Kornick C, Kramarich SS, Lamer TJ, et al. Complications of lumbar facet radiofrequency denervation. Spine 2004;29:1352–4.
38. Nath S, Nath CS, Pettersson K. Percutaneous lumbar zygapophysial(facet) joint neurotomy using radiofrequency current, in the management of chronic low back pain. Spine 2008;33:1291–7.

Safety and Complications of Cervical Epidural Steroid Injections

Byron J. Schneider, MD*, Simone Maybin, MD, Eric Sturos, MD

KEYWORDS

- Epidural injection • Interlaminar • Transforaminal • Cervical radiculopathy
- Corticosteroids • Safety • Complications

KEY POINTS

- The most common adverse events related to cervical epidural steroid injections, such as procedure-related pain and vasovagal reactions, are minor, self-limited, and not unique to this type of injection.
- The risk of neurologic damage from cervical interlaminar epidural steroid injections (CILESI) is caused by aberrant needle placement or space-occupying lesions.
- Risks of CILESI are mitigated by use of contralateral oblique technique, limiting use of sedation, injection at C6-7 or below, sterile technique, and following anticoagulation guidelines.
- The risk of neurologic damage from cervical transforaminal epidural steroid injections is caused by embolic infarct when inadvertent intra-arterial injection of particulate steroids has occurred.
- Only nonparticulate dexamethasone should be used for cervical transforaminal epidural steroid injections.

INTRODUCTION

Cervical radicular pain has an age-adjusted incidence of 83 per 100,000 people in the US population.[1] Although symptoms can vary, initially severe pain can be present. Cervical epidural steroid injections are a potential treatment option. Nearly 250,000 cervical or thoracic epidural injections were performed in the US Medicare populations in 2013.[2] There are two approaches to perform a cervical epidural steroid injection, transforaminal or interlaminar, with the interlaminar approach being nearly four times more common.[2] The most common complications related to either of these

The authors have nothing to disclose.
Department of Physical Medicine and Rehabilitation, Vanderbilt University Medical Center, 2201 Children's Way Suite 1318, Nashville, TN 37212, USA
* Corresponding author.
E-mail address: Byron.j.schneider@vanderbilt.edu

Phys Med Rehabil Clin N Am 29 (2018) 155–169
https://doi.org/10.1016/j.pmr.2017.08.012
1047-9651/18/© 2017 Elsevier Inc. All rights reserved.

approaches are common to other needle-based interventions or medications in general. These include procedure-related pain and steroid side effects.[3] That said, both approaches also have risks of more serious complications, such as neurologic damage.[4-15] Each approach is unique in the potential etiology of causing such damage, however, and accordingly risk-mitigation techniques for either approach differ. This article covers the rare but unique serious risks of neurologic damage with cervical epidural steroid injections, differentiates the risk profiles of the interlaminar and transforaminal approaches, describes the more common complications of cervical epidural steroid injections, and reviews relevant safety mitigation techniques.

CERVICAL TRANSFORAMINAL EPIDURAL STEROID INJECTIONS
Anatomy and Technique

Cervical transforaminal epidural steroid injections (CTFESI) use an anterior oblique approach and target the epidural space within the posterior inferior neuroforamen. This approach passes the needle within close proximity to several vital vascular structures that feed the central nervous system (CNS). The ascending or deep cervical arteries pass upward to the anterior tubercles of the transverse processes and can anastomosis with medullary branches that feed the spinal cord via the external foraminal opening at any level from C3-4 to C7-T1.[16] The vertebral artery is another vital vascular structure the needle is in close proximity to, which arises from the subclavian artery or ascending aorta and then typically enters the neuroforamina at C6 and then ascends ventral to the accepted target of CTFESI.[16] The vertebral artery, which feeds the brain, can give rise to segmental medullary arteries that also feed the spinal cord.

The potential to cause insult to the arterial supply of the CNS during CTFESI because of the needle's close proximity to these vital arterial structures is unique to CTFESI.

Central Nervous System Complications

Reports of quadriparesis, stroke, and even death following CTFESI began appearing in the early 2000s.[4,5,7,9,10,13,17,18] The first such report published in 2001 described a case of cervical spinal cord infarction and eventual death after CTFESI.[5] In 2003 another case of immediate cervical spinal cord infarction and death following a C6-7 TFESI was reported.[9] An additional case of cortical blindness following CTFESI was also reported in 2003.[19] At the time little was known about the mechanism of injury, although autopsy from one case showed microscopic vertebral arterial wall dissection without gross evidence of dissection.[9] Around the same time, others were beginning to suspect that inadvertent injection of particulate steroids into vulnerable arteries feeding the CNS was resulting in embolic infarcts.[18]

In 2004, another case report of quadriparesis and brainstem herniation after C5-6 TFESI was published, with the authors again suspecting injury to be a result of embolic infarct caused by inadvertent intra-arterial injection of particulate steroid preparations.[18] Despite these early concerns, particulate steroids continued to be used regularly for CTFESI. Additional reports of motor incomplete tetraplegia and cerebellar infarction appeared soon after.[4,7,13]

In a 2007 survey of more than 1000 physicians major complications following CTFESI were anonymously reported as follows: 16 cases of vertebrobasilar brain infarcts (the cerebellum, brainstem, or posterior cerebral artery territory), 12 cases of cervical spinal cord infarcts, and two combined brain/spinal cord infarcts.[10] Thirteen of these cases resulted in death. Although case reports and surveys are unable to provide a true incidence of these complications, it was clear that there was a risk of paralysis, stroke, and even death following CTFESI that warranted further explanation. In the following years, significant progress was made in better understanding why these complications were occurring and how to prevent them from occurring.

Mechanism of Injury

Initially some postulated that damage to arterial structures themselves, such as arterial spasm or arterial dissection, was the causative mechanism of injury during CTFESI.[9,20,21] However, as more was learned about the vascular anatomy, steroid particle properties, and the interplay between these via animal studies, injury caused by embolic effects of intra-arterial administration of particulate steroids became the most accepted etiology of these injuries.

Particulate steroids (methylprednisolone, betamethasone, triamcinolone) are steroid preparations that are insoluble in water and form large particles or aggregates.[22] These same properties were thought to confer a superior therapeutic effect, which is likely why particulate steroids were frequently used for CTFESI in the early 2000s. The size of methylprednisolone particles can be in excess of 50 μm.[18,23] Triamcinolone and methylprednisolone also tend to coalesce into large aggregates in excess of 100 μm.[18] Betamethasone particles, although extremely small individually, densely pack together forming aggregates with sizes greater than 100 μm.[22] These are all significantly larger than a 6- to 8-μm red blood cell (RBC), which is just small enough to pass through a capillary.[22]

Several vital vascular structures may be encountered during CTFESI. In fact, a cadaveric study found that in 21 of 95 cervical foramina dissected, the ascending, deep cervical, or other major arterial branch was proximal to the posterior aspect of the foraminal opening and within 2 mm of the needle path during CTFESI.[24] Of those 21 locations, seven actually formed an anastomosis with a feeding medullary artery entering the foramen at the respective level. In addition to this, the vertebral artery is present within the neuroforamen at C6 and higher.[16]

Animal studies provided further in vivo evidence that intra-arterial injection of particulate steroids results in embolic infarct because of steroid occlusion or RBC aggregate occlusion.[25] One study performed direct injection of steroids into the vertebral artery of pigs. It showed that the group injected with methylprednisolone resulted in permanent neurologic hypoxic/ischemic damage.[26] Similarly, direct injection of particulate steroids into the carotid artery of rats has also been found to cause permanent neurologic injury.[18,23,25,27]

Fortunately, this same body of evidence consistently reported on the relative safety of the nonparticulate steroid dexamethasone. Dexamethasone is smaller than the size of an RBC, with particles only 0.5 μm in size.[22] Dexamethasone has also been shown to not result in spiculated RBC aggregate formation.[25] Animal studies have then shown that intra-arterial injection of dexamethasone into swine or mice does not cause neurologic injury.[18,23,25–27] Given this information, it is not surprising that all cases of neurologic infarct following CTFESI have used particulate steroid preparations, with no such complications being reported when dexamethasone is used for CTFESI.

However, a recent report was published of spinal cord (conus medullaris) infarct following lumbar transforaminal injection using dexamethasone.[28] Although the full implications of this report are unclear, this suggests that other mechanisms of injury are also possible. Two recent studies found that if dexamethasone is mixed with ropivacaine, it can result in a rapid pH-dependent crystallization reaction that forms precipitates of unsafe size.[29,30] It is possible other factors may also result in dexamethasone crystallization. Arterial vasospasm or dissections have also been considered as potential causes.[9,20,21]

Safety Techniques

In response to the Food and Drug Administration warnings of neurologic damage after epidural steroid injections and requiring label changes,[17] a Multisociety Pain Workgroup composed of 13 different medical societies was formed. In 2015 the Multisociety Pain Workgroup published opinions regarding CTFESI, unanimously stating that particulate steroids should not be used in CFTESI and only the nonparticulate steroid dexamethasone be used.[31] Even if using dexamethasone, however, other safety techniques that minimize the risk of inadvertent intra-arterial needle placement and subsequent steroid injection should also be followed.

Technical aspects are used to minimize the risk of positioning the needle within an artery. The needle should be positioned within the lateral portion of the posterior inferior the foramen, immediately adjacent to the superior articular process.[32] This minimizes the chance of injecting the vertebral artery, which is located in the anterior portion of the foramen. This needles position also limits the risk of injecting into radicular arteries, which tend to run above or in front of the spinal nerve.[32,33]

The use of imaging with real-time contrast is also vital to recognize vascular contrast patterns. Although computed tomography (CT)-guided CTFESI has been described,[34] the use of fluoroscopy is much more common. Fluoroscopy identifies vascular uptake patterns 19.6% of the time.[35] Rates are similar (26%) if CT guidance is used.[36] There is no reliable way to differentiate between venous and arterial uptake, and as such all vascular flow must be assumed to be potentially arterial.

Other methods have been developed to detect vascular uptake that may be missed by imaging with real-time contrast administration. Digital subtraction angiography is a tool that enhances visualization of contrast flow patterns by subtracting pixel values of an initial scout image from subsequent images obtained during live contrast administration.[37] In one study, intravascular injection was detected in 17.9% of CTFESIs performed without digital subtraction angiography versus 32.8% when digital subtraction angiography was used ($P = .0471$).[38] Another study later confirmed that digital subtraction angiography statistically increases the ability to detect vascular uptake compared with traditional fluoroscopy.[39]

Use of an anesthetic test dose can also detect vascular uptake missed by imaging.[40,41] By injecting a local anesthetic first, such symptoms as acute onset dizziness, tachycardia, metallic taste, full-body paresthesias, auditory changes, slurred speech, and motor ataxia or even temporary paralysis and seizure are induced if the needle is located within an artery.[42] In severe cases, inadvertently administration of lidocaine into a cervical artery has even resulted in cardiovascular sequelae and/or death.[40,43,44] The overall incidence of a positive anesthetic test dose during CTFESI is 0.59%.[41] When performing an anesthetic test dose, ropivacaine should not be used.[29,30] The risks and benefits of the anesthetic test dose should be weighed carefully, and careful consideration should be given as to whether an anesthetic test dose is needed if nonparticulate steroid is administered.[45]

Multiple safety techniques now exist to detect when the needle has inadvertently been placed within a vascular structure. Moreover, adopting the use of dexamethasone seems to have greatly reduced the risk of inadvertent intra-arterial injections that result in neurologic damage. These significant advances seem to have made CTFESI safer. The only recent reports of neurologic injury have been from improper use of imaging resulting in the needle penetrating the spinal cord itself,[46] or continued use of particulate steroids.[47] There are no current reports of neurologic injury occurring when CTFESI has been performed in accordance with current standards of care.

CERVICAL INTERLAMINAR EPIDURAL STEROID INJECTIONS
Technical Descriptions and Anatomic Considerations

Cervical interlaminar epidural steroid injections (CILESI) also carry the risk of paralysis,[6,8,11,14,48–50] although this risk differs because of different anatomic considerations. An interlaminar approach uses a midline or paramidline approach posteriorly and targets the epidural space between the dura anteriorly and ligamentum flavum posteriorly. The target for the needle tip is within a few millimeters of the spinal canal. Advancement of the needle too anteriorly can result in dural puncture and potentially cord penetration. The target space is also confined by the posterior spinal column. This introduces the risk of space-occupying lesions, such as epidural hematoma or epidural abscess, which have the potential to compress the spinal cord.

Major Complications

Aberrant needle placement

Even with ideal needle placement during CILESI, the needle is within millimeters of the thecal sac. Inherently, this poses the risk of inadvertent needle placement into the thecal sac or spinal cord. This complication is compounded if unrecognized and certain medications are subsequently administered.

If intrathecal placement is identified before medications are administered, the primary risk is spinal headache. If intrathecal administration of iodine-based contrast, such as iopamidol (Isovue) or iohexol (Omnipaque) occurs, the added risk is minimal because such forms of contrast are approved for intrathecal use for procedures, such as CT myelogram. However, there are additional risks if gadolinium-based contrast is being used. Gadolinium-based contrasts are not Food and Drug Administration approved for intrathecal use, and reports of gadolinium encephalopathy after intrathecal administration of gadolinium exist.[51] If intrathecal needle placement and intrathecal contrast administration are unrecognized, intrathecal steroid or anesthetic administration may also occur. There have been reported cases of arachnoiditis after intrathecal administration of various steroid preparations.[52–54] Cervical intrathecal administration of anesthetic also poses a high risk of high spinal anesthesia, which could result in respiratory failure requiring ventilation.

The risk of neurologic damage caused by inadvertent needle placement occurs if the needle is placed into the spinal cord itself. The first reported cases of spinal cord injury during CILESI from direct spinal cord trauma involved patients who were given intravenous sedation and underwent C5-6 ILESI.[6] In each case, the sedated patient was unable to demonstrate signs of pain or irritation when the spinal cord was penetrated. One patient acutely developed severe pain, paresthesia, and weakness on the right in a C7 and C8 distribution and right thigh paresthesias and did not experience significant recovery. The other patient acutely developed severe left arm pain and right thigh paresthesia that evolved into severe refractory reflex sympathetic dystrophy of the left arm. In both cases, MRI revealed signs of intrinsic spinal cord damage at the level of injection.[6] A recent case shared similar characteristics.[50] The patient underwent a C5-6 CILESI while under intravenous sedation and acutely developed severe neck pain, right facial paresthesia, and right arm and leg weakness and numbness on awakening from sedation. The patient had persistent motor deficits. MRI again revealed evidence of intrinsic spinal cord damage.[50] Two additional reports of motor incomplete cervical spinal cord injuries following cervical epidural steroid injections seem to be a result of aberrant needle placement into the spinal cord during CILESI, although details are limited.[11] One case resulted in a patient suffering C2 American Spinal Injury Association Impairment Scale Spinal Cord Injury (AIS SCI) with predominantly left-sided weakness after intraparenchymal contrast administration. In the other case, the patient was reported to suffer a "spinal contusion" after an "interventional spine procedure," resulting in C6 AIS SCI.[11]

Safety Techniques

The available case reports highlight two important safety considerations, because in three of these, complications occurred after sedated patients underwent C5-6 CILESI.[6,50] The natural bulge in the mid-portion of the cervical spinal cord places the spinal cord in even closer proximity to the epidural space and further reduces the margin of error. Because of the cervicogenic bulge, current recommendations are that CILESI only be performed at C6-7 or below.[31] With injection at more caudal levels, adequate medications spread can still be achieved. With 5 mL of injectate, injection at C7-T1 results in medication spread up to C5-6 100% of the time.[55] Because of the use of sedation in these reports, patients were unable to report pain or irritation when the needle encountered the spinal cord. For this reason, another recommendation is that routine use of sedation for CILESI should be avoided.[32] Moreover, in rare cases when intravenous sedation is used, it would reason that only minimal doses required to achieve anxiolysis be used, so that a patient can still respond to and report symptoms that may indicate the needle is encroaching on the spinal cord.

Accurate visualization of the needle tip can also aid in avoiding aberrant needle placement into the thecal sac or spinal cord, which is best achieved with the use of a contralateral oblique approach.[56] Gauging needle depth via a lateral fluoroscopic view during CILESI is frequently complicated by the view being obstructed by the shoulders. Moreover, any deviation from a true midline approach results in the needle tip appearing deeper than the target space before the epidural space is encountered. By using a contralateral oblique fluoroscopic view that matches the obliquity of the cervical lamina, a true radiologic landmark formed by the interlaminar line is achieved that can be used to accurately ascertain needle depth. Moreover, this approach negates geometric amplification of needle depth when it is off of midline.[56,57] Since development of this technique, additional research has shown that a contralateral oblique view of 50° is optimal for minimizing the risk of passing the needle too far.[57]

To best mitigate the risk of aberrant needle location during CILESI, the use of intravenous sedation should be avoided, injections should not be performed above the C6-7 level, and the contralateral oblique technique during multiplanar fluoroscopic imaging should be used.

Epidural Abscess

Cervical epidural abscess following CILESI with resulting spinal cord compression is a rare but serious complication. Only a limited number of case reports exist. In one case, the patient presented 72 hours after CILESI with shaking chills and a stiff neck. After CT myelography revealed a C3-T1 epidural abscess, he underwent emergent decompression. Cultures were positive for *Staphylococcus aureus*. The patient did regain the ability to ambulate without an assistive device but had persistent motor incomplete quadriparesis.[14] In the other fully described case of epidural abscess after CILESI, the patient presented with increased axial neck pain and chills 7 days after injection. Antibiotics were not started until leukocytosis was found on Day 15 postinjection. Still 1 week later the patient developed left arm pain, paresthesia, and weakness, at which point MRI demonstrated epidural abscess from C4-C6. He then underwent decompressive laminectomy. Intraoperative cultures were positive for *S aureus*. By 7 months he had returned to baseline neurologic function.[49] There are two additional cases with limited details that also seem to be of epidural abscess following CILESI with persistent motor incomplete spinal cord injuries despite surgical decompression.[11] Cervical epidural abscess following CILESI is a rare complication, with initial symptoms of pain and subjective fever presenting days after injection before neurologic deficits appear. High clinical suspicion is warranted, because proper treatment including surgical decompression and debridement along with antibiotics can result in partial or complete resolution of neurologic deficits.

The risks of epidural abscess are mitigated by proper use of aseptic technique. Current Spine Intervention Society guidelines recommend sterile preparation be performed with 2% chlorhexidine in 70% alcohol.[32] This solution has been found to be superior to iodine-based solutions for prevention of surgical infections[58] and has been found to be safe for spinal anesthesia.[59] The use of face masks is also recommended when performing spinal injection procedures, because they have been shown to be effective in limiting spread of oropharyngeal droplets.[60,61] Sterile gloves should also be used.[32]

Epidural Hematoma

Another rare but serious complication following CILESI is epidural or subdural hematoma with resulting spinal cord compression. The first reported case was of a patient that presented with difficulty passing urine 2 hours after C7-T1 ILESI.[15] The patient was on indomethacin at the time of the injection. Symptoms progressed to flaccid paralysis of both lower extremities and sensory deficits. He demonstrated recovery of neurologic deficits, with exception of urinary retention, after laminectomy and evacuation of a C7-T3 hematoma.[15] A similar case involved a patient on diclofenac, clopidogrel, and possibly aspirin who underwent CILESI and developed weakness and numbness in all four extremities 30 minutes after injection.[48] He had recovery of the upper extremities but remained paraplegic despite emergent C3-T3 laminectomy and hematoma evacuation.[48] An additional case reported persistent motor incomplete paraplegia (T2 AIS C) despite surgical decompression following what seems to be CILESI while on "anticoagulation."[11] In all three of these cases, the patient was on some form of antiplatelet or anticoagulation medication and experienced persistence of some neurologic deficits despite surgical decompression.

There has been at least one report of death as a result of CILESI complicated by epidural hematoma. A 62-year-old woman who underwent C4-5 CILESI acutely developed neck and shoulder pain, paresthesias, and progressive weakness over the course of hours. Despite emergent surgical evacuation of a C2-6 subdural hematoma, she remained hemiplegic on the right. Unfortunately, postoperative course was complicated by meningitis and she ultimately died because of cardiopulmonary arrest.[8]

There is an additional case of persistent sensory deficit following epidural hematoma. A patient who had recently stopped ibuprofen underwent C5-6 CILESI and then presented with an acute Brown-Séquard syndrome 8 days postinjection, although cervical manipulation had also been done the day before symptom onset. After successful laminectomy, his only persistent neurologic symptoms was persistent numbness from C3-C7.[12]

There are additional cases of epidural hematoma following CILESI that demonstrated complete resolution of symptoms following surgical decompression. In one case, a patient on diclofenac presented with right-sided hemiplegia, left-sided sensory deficits, bowel and bladder incontinence, and right-sided Horner syndrome 30 minutes after C6-7 CILESI. Symptoms resolved after C6-T2 laminectomy.[62] In another case, the patient presented with neck pain and Brown-Séquard syndrome deficits 2 hours after C7-T1 ILESI and experienced complete recovery after C3-C7 laminectomy.[63] Lastly, a patient developed severe neck pain and upper extremity paresthesias

10 minutes after C7-T1 CILESI and experienced full recovery after emergent C4-T3 laminectomy. Of note, clopidogrel was stopped 12 days before the injection.[64]

Even with ideal technique, the risk of epidural hematoma and possible spinal cord compression exists any time CILESI is performed. Symptom onset can be acute, but may also present days later. Because of this, physicians must educate patients on symptoms to be wary of, such as worsening pain and weakness or numbness in any of the extremities. In some of the previously mentioned cases, emergent recognition of the hematoma and subsequent surgical evacuation and decompression resulted in symptom resolution.

Although the risk of hematoma is always present, there are factors that can exacerbate this. In the lumbar spine there have been reported cases of epidural hematoma after ILESI in patients with undiagnosed bleeding disorders.[65,66] If patients report symptoms that may be suggestive of such disorders, consider further working this up before injection is made.

The risk of hematoma may also be increased by various medications. The current American Society of Regional Anesthesia guidelines stratify CILESI steroid injections as an intermediate-risk procedure.[67] Per this classification, all anticoagulation, such as heparin, low-molecular-weight heparin, and warfarin, must be stopped before CILESI. P2Y12 inhibitors, such as clopidogrel, should also be stopped. Aspirin is recommended to be continued or stopped based on "shared assessment and risk stratification with the patient." Nonsteroidal anti-inflammatory drugs (NSAIDs) do not need to be stopped, nor does cilostazol or dipyrimadole.[67] Some have suggested these guidelines indiscriminately lump CILESI together with other spine-based procedures that have a much lower risk profile of a spinal cord compression because of hematoma, and that further caution may be warranted.[68] For example, there are no known reports of epidural hematoma causing neurologic damage after transforaminal epidural injections, medial branch blocks, or sacroiliac joint injections. This is clearly in contrast to the risk of bleeding after CILESI.

Early anesthesia-based literature reported that the incidence of epidural hematoma after accessing the lumbar epidural space via an interlaminar approach for epidural blocks was 1 in 150,000.[69] In a more recent study, 1 in 2026 (0.05%; 95% confidence interval, 0.00–0.31) ILESI resulted in hematoma in patients not on antiplatelet or anticoagulation medications. Of note, this occurred after lumbar ILESI. No ILESI in this study were performed on patients on antiplatelet or anticoagulation medications.[70] Presumably, given the physiologic effects of antiplatelet or anticoagulation medications, the risk of epidural hematoma while on these medication would be, at best, not statistically different and at worst much higher. Based on these results, the authors proposed a modified 2013 Spine Intervention Society–2015 American Society of Regional Anesthesia guideline table that placed ILESI in an "intermediate-high" category. Changes include that consideration should be made to stopping NSAIDs for five half-lives before ILESI and that cilostazol or dipyridamole be stopped before ILESI.[70] Aspirin continued to have a "shared decision-making" status for ILESI.[70] Although this represents a slightly more conservative approach to stopping certain medications before ILESI, the physician is still required to make an informed decision with respect to NSAIDs or aspirin.

The physician then must balance the risks of continuing medications, such as aspirin or NSAIDS, which have antiplatelet effect before ILESI and the possibility that this increases the risk of epidural hematoma against the risk of stopping these medications. In one study that specifically reported on complications related to continuing or stopping anticoagulant or antiplatelet medications for interventional spine procedures, 701 cases had antiplatelet medications held and no cardiovascular or cerebrovascular complications occurred.[71] In a similar study, 1676 cases had antiplatelet medications held for interventional spine procedures, again without cardiovascular or cerebrovascular complication noted.[72] In total this represents a complication rate related to holding antiplatelet medications for interventional spine procedures of 0 in 2377 (0%; 95% confidence interval, 0%–0.001%).[73] Alternatively, there are likely times where stopping such medications may be contraindicated. What is clear, however, is that although the risk of epidural hematoma after ILESI is low even while on medications, such as aspirin, the risk of stopping these medications temporarily is also extremely low.

OTHER ADVERSE EVENTS
Common Adverse Events

The adverse events following cervical epidural steroid injection that are most likely to be encountered clinically tend to be minor, often self-limited, and are common to other forms of medication administration or needle-based procedures. The largest published cohort that tracked adverse events after epidural steroid injection evaluated more than 16,000 epidural steroid injections and found that the overall incidence of immediate adverse events was 2.4% and delayed adverse events was 4.9%.[3] The most common of these were central steroid response (2.6%), increased pain (2.1%), and vasovagal reactions (1.2%).[3] There were no reports of serious complications in this large cohort, and all other reported adverse events occurred with a frequency of less than 1%. No significant associations were found with respect to the spinal segment (cervical vs thoracic vs lumbar) or approach (interlaminar vs transforaminal) in the frequency of any of the minor adverse events reported, with the exception of dural punctures occurring more frequently in interlaminar injections.[3]

Steroid Side Effects

The side effect of central steroid response (2.6%) represents a side effect of the steroid medication itself and is not unique to steroid injections.[3] Symptoms of central steroid effect include facial flushing and nonpositional headaches.[74] Although unpleasant, these symptoms are not dangerous and are self-limited with duration of hours to days.

Potentially more serious adverse events related to steroid are the potential endocrinologic effects. Patients with diabetes can reasonably expect a temporary elevation of blood glucose of 100 mg/dL or more for approximately 48 to 72 hours after an epidural steroid injection.[75,76] This response has been found to be dose dependent.[77] In patients without diabetes, there may be subclinical effects on insulin sensitivity but effects on blood glucose levels are much less common.[78,79] However, steroid-induced hyperglycemia can occur with all forms of exogenous corticosteroids.[80]

Other steroid-related side effects after epidural steroid administration have also been reported. Multiple studies have found that suppression of the hypothalamic-pituitary axis occurs for an average of 21 days.[79,81,82] Clinicians can reasonable expect hypothalamic-pituitary axis suppression to be asymptomatic, however, unless other systemic stresses are concomitant. Hypothalamic-pituitary axis suppression is a well-recognized phenomenon that occurs with other forms of steroid administration.[83]

There are reports of decreased bone density associated with greater than 10 epidural steroid injections, a known side effect of systemic corticosteroids.[84] Other studies that investigated women exposed to fewer injections have failed to corroborate this.[85] Conflicting evidence also exists as it relates to potential temporary increases in blood pressure after epidural steroid injections.[86] Rarely, other systemic effects, such as abnormal vaginal bleeding, epidural lipomatosis, visual deficits, and transient Cushing syndrome, have also been reported after epidural administration of steroid.[87–91]

To best mitigate these adverse events caused by steroids, the physician should limit cumulative exposure to steroids. Patients at risk of these complications, including patients with diabetes or adrenal insufficiency, should also be identified as being at increased risk.

Contrast Side Effects

The use of real-time fluoroscopy with contrast is vital to safely performing cervical epidural steroid injections. Accordingly adverse events related to administration of the contrast itself are a possibility. In general, 0.7% to 3.1% of patients will have mild immediate reactions to nonionic iodinated contrast.[92,93] If an allergy to contrast is known, the physician may elect to premedicate depending on the severity of the allergy. This is done with 32 mg oral methylprednisolone 12 and 2 hours before the procedure, with the option of also administering 50 mg diphenhydramine.[94] Even with premedication, there can be up to an 18% chance of a breakthrough reaction, of which 1.6% is severe.[95]

Another alternative is the use of gadolinium-based contrast. In a chart review of 127 patients with allergy to iodinated contrast who then had spinal procedures done with gadolinium-based contrast, no complications were noted.[96] In general, severe allergy to gadolinium-based contrast is extremely rare. However, in patients with severe renal failure, nephrogenic systemic sclerosis is a possibility.[97]

SUMMARY

The risk of serious neurologic complications following CILESI and CTFESI is extremely low but definitively not zero.[3] All reports of such complications exist in case report form only. Evidence strongly suggests that the risk of infarcting the spinal cord or posterior brain structures during CTFESI is caused by the embolic effect of inadvertent arterial injection of particulate steroids.[18,23,25,27] Only using the nonparticulate steroid dexamethasone in CTFESI best mitigates this risk. The risk of neurologic damage from CILESI is caused by either aberrant needle placement or mass lesions, such as epidural hematoma or abscess. Use of proper imaging techniques, following anticoagulation guidelines, and proper sterile technique can limit but not eliminate these risks. The most common adverse events that occur following CTFESI or CILESI are procedural-related pain, steroid side effects, and vasovagal reactions.[3] These are minor, self-limited, and not unique to cervical epidural steroid injections.[3] Other treatment options, such as oral medications and surgery, similarly have risks that must also be considered when determining a treatment plan for cervical radicular pain. When performed properly, the judicious use of cervical epidural steroid injection to treat cervical radicular pain remains a safe and viable treatment option.

REFERENCES

1. Radhakrishnan K, Litchy WJ, O'Fallon WM, et al. Epidemiology of cervical radiculopathy. A population-based study from Rochester, Minnesota, 1976 through 1990. Brain 1994;117(Pt 2):325–35.
2. Manchikanti L, Hirsch JA. Neurological complications associated with epidural steroid injections. Curr Pain Headache Rep 2015;19(5):482.

3. El-Yahchouchi CA, Plastaras CT, Maus TP, et al. Adverse event rates associated with transforaminal and interlaminar epidural steroid injections: a multi-institutional study. Pain Med 2016;17(2):239–49.
4. Beckman WA, Mendez RJ, Paine GF, et al. Cerebellar herniation after cervical transforaminal epidural injection. Reg Anesth Pain Med 2006;31(3):282–5.
5. Brouwers PJ, Kottink EJ, Simon MA, et al. A cervical anterior spinal artery syndrome after diagnostic blockade of the right C6-nerve root. Pain 2001;91(3): 397–9.
6. Hodges SD, Castleberg RL, Miller T, et al. Cervical epidural steroid injection with intrinsic spinal cord damage. Two case reports. Spine 1998;23(19): 2137–42, 2142.
7. Ludwig MA, Burns SP. Spinal cord infarction following cervical transforaminal epidural injection: a case report. Spine 2005;30(10):E266–8.
8. Reitman CA, Watters W. Subdural hematoma after cervical epidural steroid injection. Spine 2002;27(6):E174–6.
9. Rozin L, Rozin R, Koehler SA, et al. Death during transforaminal epidural steroid nerve root block (C7) due to perforation of the left vertebral artery. Am J Forensic Med Pathol 2003;24(4):351–5.
10. Scanlon GC, Moeller-Bertram T, Romanowsky SM, et al. Cervical transforaminal epidural steroid injections: more dangerous than we think? Spine 2007;32(11): 1249–56.
11. Schreiber AL, McDonald BP, Kia F, et al. Cervical epidural steroid injections and spinal cord injuries. Spine J 2015;16(10):1163–6.
12. Stoll A, Sanchez M. Epidural hematoma after epidural block: implications for its use in pain management. Surg Neurol 2002;57(4):235–40.
13. Suresh S, Berman J, Connell DA. Cerebellar and brainstem infarction as a complication of CT-guided transforaminal cervical nerve root block. Skeletal Radiol 2007;36(5):449–52.
14. Waldman SD. Cervical epidural abscess after cervical epidural nerve block with steroids. Anesth Analg 1991;72(5):717–8.
15. Williams KN, Jackowski A, Evans PJ. Epidural haematoma requiring surgical decompression following repeated cervical epidural steroid injections for chronic pain. Pain 1990;42(2):197–9.
16. Gillilan LA. The arterial blood supply of the human spinal cord. J Comp Neurol 1958;110(1):75–103.
17. Research, C. for D. E. and. (n.d.). Drug safety and availability - FDA Drug Safety Communication: FDA requires label changes to warn of rare but serious neurologic problems after epidural corticosteroid injections for pain. Available at: http://www.fda.gov/Drugs/DrugSafety/ucm394280.htm. Accessed March 1, 2016.
18. Tiso RL, Cutler T, Catania JA, et al. Adverse central nervous system sequelae after selective transforaminal block: the role of corticosteroids. Spine J 2004;4(4): 468–74.
19. McMillan MR, Crumpton C. Cortical blindness and neurologic injury complicating cervical transforaminal injection for cervical radiculopathy. Anesthesiology 2003; 99(2):509–11.
20. Wallace MA, Fukui MB, Williams RL, et al. Complications of cervical selective nerve root blocks performed with fluoroscopic guidance. AJR Am J Roentgenol 2007;188(5):1218–21.
21. Ziai WC, Ardelt AA, Llinas RH. Brainstem stroke following uncomplicated cervical epidural steroid injection. Arch Neurol 2006;63(11):1643.

22. Derby R, Lee S-H, Date ES, et al. Size and aggregation of corticosteroids used for epidural injections. Pain Med 2008;9(2):227–34.
23. Benzon HT, Chew T-L, McCarthy RJ, et al. Comparison of the particle sizes of different steroids and the effect of dilution: a review of the relative neurotoxicities of the steroids. Anesthesiology 2007;106(2):331–8.
24. Huntoon MA. Anatomy of the cervical intervertebral foramina: vulnerable arteries and ischemic neurologic injuries after transforaminal epidural injections. Pain 2005;117(1):104–11.
25. Laemmel E, Segal N, Mirshahi M, et al. Deleterious effects of intra-arterial administration of particulate steroids on microvascular perfusion in a mouse model. Radiology 2016;279(3):731–40.
26. Okubadejo GO, Talcott MR, Schmidt RE, et al. Perils of intravascular methylprednisolone injection into the vertebral artery. An animal study. J Bone Joint Surg Am 2008;90(9):1932–8.
27. Dawley JD, Moeller-Bertram T, Wallace MS, et al. Intra-arterial injection in the rat brain: evaluation of steroids used for transforaminal epidurals. Spine 2009;34(16):1638–43.
28. Gharibo CG, Fakhry M, Diwan S, et al. Conus medullaris infarction after a right L4 transforaminal epidural steroid injection using dexamethasone. Pain Physician 2016;19(8):E1211–4.
29. Hwang H, Park J, Lee WK, et al. Crystallization of local anesthetics when mixed with corticosteroid solutions. Ann Rehabil Med 2016;40(1):21.
30. Watkins TW, Dupre S, Coucher JR. Ropivacaine and dexamethasone: a potentially dangerous combination for therapeutic pain injections. J Med Imaging Radiat Oncol 2015;59(5):571–7.
31. Rathmell JP, Benzon HT, Dreyfuss P, et al. Safeguards to prevent neurologic complications after epidural steroid injections: consensus opinions from a multidisciplinary Working Group and National Organizations. Anesthesiology 2015;122(5):974–84.
32. Bogduk N. Practice guidelines for spinal diagnostic and treatment procedures. 2nd edition. San Francisco: International Spine Intervention Society; 2013.
33. Hoeft MA, Rathmell JP, Monsey RD, et al. Cervical transforaminal injection and the radicular artery: variation in anatomical location within the cervical intervertebral foramina. Reg Anesth Pain Med 2006;31(3):270–4.
34. Wald JT, Maus TP, Geske JR, et al. Safety and efficacy of CT-guided transforaminal cervical epidural steroid injections using a posterior approach. AJNR Am J Neuroradiol 2012;33(3):415–9.
35. Furman MB, Giovanniello MT, O'Brien EM. Incidence of intravascular penetration in transforaminal cervical epidural steroid injections. Spine 2003;28(1):21–5.
36. Kranz PG, Raduazo P, Gray L, et al. CT fluoroscopy-guided cervical interlaminar steroid injections: safety, technique, and radiation dose parameters. AJNR Am J Neuroradiol 2012;33(7):1221–4.
37. Jasper JF. Role of digital subtraction fluoroscopic imaging in detecting intravascular injections. Pain Physician 2003;6(3):369–72.
38. McLean JP, Sigler JD, Plastaras CT, et al. The rate of detection of intravascular injection in cervical transforaminal epidural steroid injections with and without digital subtraction angiography. PM&R 2009;1(7):636–42.
39. Rubens A, Pino C, Ivie C. Utility of digital subtraction angiography in cervical transforaminal epidural steroid injections: does digital subtraction improve safety over live fluoroscopy? 14th Annual Pain Medicine Meeting. Miami, Florida, November 2015.
40. Karasek M, Bogduk N. Temporary neurologic deficit after cervical transforaminal injection of local anesthetic. Pain Med 2004;5(2):202–5.

41. Smuck M, Maxwell MD, Kennedy D, et al. Utility of the anesthetic test dose to avoid catastrophic injury during cervical transforaminal epidural injections. Spine J 2010;10(10):857–64.

42. Kennedy DJ, Dreyfuss P, Aprill CN, et al. Paraplegia following image-guided transforaminal lumbar spine epidural steroid injection: two case reports. Pain Med 2009;10(8):1389–94.

43. Chung SG. Convulsion caused by a lidocaine test in cervical transforaminal epidural steroid injection. PM&R 2011;3(7):674–7.

44. Mahli A, Coskun D, Akcali DT. Aetiology of convulsions due to stellate ganglion block: a review and report of two cases. Eur J Anaesthesiol 2002;19(5):376–80.

45. DeFrancesch F, O'Brien D, Smith C. Anesthetic test dose and seizure risk with cervical transforaminal epidural steroid injection. Spine Intervention Society. 2017. Available at: https://c.ymcdn.com/sites/www.spineintervention.org/resource/resmgr/factfinder/FactFinder_2017-05-01_Test_D.pdf. Accessed July 11, 207.

46. Lee J-H, Lee J-K, Seo B-R, et al. Spinal cord injury produced by direct damage during cervical transforaminal epidural injection. Reg Anesth Pain Med 2008; 33(4):377–9.

47. Moon J, Kwon H-M. Spinal cord infarction after cervical transforaminal epidural steroid injection: case report and literature review. Case Rep Neurol 2017;9:1–5.

48. Benzon HT, Wong HY, Siddiqui T, et al. Caution in performing epidural injections in patients on several antiplatelet drugs. Anesthesiology 1999;91(5):1558–9.

49. Huang RC, Shapiro GS, Lim M, et al. Cervical epidural abscess after epidural steroid injection. Spine 2004;29(1):E7–9.

50. Maddela R, Wahezi SE, Sparr S, et al. Hemiparesis and facial sensory loss following cervical epidural steroid injection. Pain Physician 2014;17(6):E761–7.

51. Kapoor R, Liu J, Devasenapathy A, et al. Gadolinium encephalopathy after intrathecal gadolinium injection. Pain Physician 2010;13(5):E321–6.

52. Abram SE, O'Connor TC. Complications associated with epidural steroid injections. Reg Anesth 1996;21(2):149–62.

53. Goldstein NP, McGuckin WF, McKenzie BF, et al. Experimental intrathecal administration of methylprednisolone acetate in multiple sclerosis. Trans Am Neurol Assoc 1970;95:243–4.

54. Nelson DA, Vates TS, Thomas RB. Complications from intrathecal steroid therapy in patients with multiple sclerosis. Acta Neurol Scand 1973;49(2):176–88.

55. Lee SE, Joe HB, Park JH, et al. Distribution range of cervical interlaminar epidural injections: a comparative study with 2.5 mL, 5 mL, and 10 mL of contrast. Pain Physician 2013;16(2):155–64.

56. Landers MH, Dreyfuss P, Bogduk N. On the geometry of fluoroscopy views for cervical interlaminar epidural injections. Pain Med 2012;13(1):58–65.

57. Gill J, Nagda J, Aner M, et al. Cervical epidural contrast spread patterns in fluoroscopic antero-posterior, lateral, and contralateral oblique view: a three-dimensional analysis. Pain Med 2017;18(6):1027–39.

58. Darouiche RO, Wall MJ, Itani KMF, et al. Chlorhexidine-alcohol versus povidone-iodine for surgical-site antisepsis. N Engl J Med 2010;362(1):18–26.

59. Sviggum HP, Jacob AK, Arendt KW, et al. Neurologic complications after chlorhexidine antisepsis for spinal anesthesia. Reg Anesth Pain Med 2012;37(2): 139–44.

60. Philips BJ, Fergusson S, Armstrong P, et al. Surgical face masks are effective in reducing bacterial contamination caused by dispersal from the upper airway. Br J Anaesth 1992;69(4):407–8.

61. Siegel J, Rhinehard E, Jackson M, et al. Guideline for isolation precautions: preventing transmission of infectious agents in healthcare settings. Healthcare Infection Control Practices Advisory Committee. Available at: https://www.cdc.gov/hicpac/pdf/isolation/isolation2007.pdf. Accessed July 11, 207.

62. Ghaly RF. Recovery after high-dose methylprednisolone and delayed evacuation: a case of spinal epidural hematoma. J Neurosurg Anesthesiol 2001;13(4):323–8.

63. Yagi S, Hida K, Iwasaki Y, et al. Cervical epidural hematoma caused by cervical twisting after epidural anesthesia: a case report. No Shinkei Geka 1998;26(7): 627–32 [in Japanese].

64. Benyamin RM, Vallejo R, Wang V, et al. Acute epidural hematoma formation in cervical spine after interlaminar epidural steroid injection despite discontinuation of Clopidogrel. Reg Anesth Pain Med 2016;41(3):398–401.

65. Yokota S, Hirabayashi Y, Wakata M, et al. Mild hemophilia A diagnosed at the onset of acute epidural hematoma after lumbar epidural block. Rinsho Ketsueki 2011;52(2):78–83 [in Japanese].

66. Yoo HS, Park SW, Han JH, et al. Paraplegia caused by an epidural hematoma in a patient with unrecognized chronic idiopathic thrombocytopenic purpura following an epidural steroid injection. Spine 2009;34(10):E376–9.

67. Narouze S, Benzon HT, Provenzano DA, et al. Interventional spine and pain procedures in patients on antiplatelet and anticoagulant medications: guidelines from the American Society of Regional Anesthesia and Pain Medicine, the European Society of Regional Anaesthesia and Pain Therapy, the American Academy of Pain Medicine, the International Neuromodulation Society, the North American Neuromodulation Society, and the World Institute of Pain. Reg Anesth Pain Med 2015;40(3):182–212.

68. Schneider B, Zheng P, Mattie R, et al. Safety of epidural steroid injections. Expert Opin Drug Saf 2016;15(8):1031–9.

69. Tryba M. Epidural regional anesthesia and low molecular heparin: pro. Anasthesiol Intensivmed Notfallmed Schmerzther 1993;28(3):179–81.

70. Goodman BS, House LM, Vallabhaneni S, et al. Anticoagulant and antiplatelet management for spinal procedures: a prospective, descriptive study and interpretation of guidelines. Pain Med 2017;18(7):1218–24.

71. Endres S, Shufelt A, Bogduk N. The risks of continuing or discontinuing anticoagulants for patients undergoing common interventional pain procedures. Pain Med 2017;18(3):403–9.

72. Manchikanti L, Malla Y, Wargo BW, et al. A prospective evaluation of bleeding risk of interventional techniques in chronic pain. Pain Physician 2011;14(4):317–29.

73. Schneider B, Maybin S. Safety and risk mitigation for cervical interlaminar epidural steroid injections. Curr Phys Med Rehabil Rep 2017.

74. Liu D, Ahmet A, Ward L, et al. A practical guide to the monitoring and management of the complications of systemic corticosteroid therapy. Allergy Asthma Clin Immunol 2013;9(1):30.

75. Even JL, Crosby CG, Song Y, et al. Effects of epidural steroid injections on blood glucose levels in patients with diabetes mellitus. Spine 2012;37(1):E46–50.

76. Gonzalez P, Laker SR, Sullivan W, et al. The effects of epidural betamethasone on blood glucose in patients with diabetes mellitus. PM&R 2009;1(4):340–5.

77. Kim WH, Sim WS, Shin BS, et al. Effects of two different doses of epidural steroid on blood glucose levels and pain control in patients with diabetes mellitus. Pain Physician 2013;16(6):557–68.

78. Ward A, Watson J, Wood P, et al. Glucocorticoid epidural for sciatica: metabolic and endocrine sequelae. Rheumatology (Oxford) 2002;41(1):68–71.

79. Younes M, Neffati F, Touzi M, et al. Systemic effects of epidural and intra-articular glucocorticoid injections in diabetic and non-diabetic patients. Joint Bone Spine 2007;74(5):472–6.

80. Tamez-Pérez HE. Steroid hyperglycemia: prevalence, early detection and therapeutic recommendations: a narrative review. World J Diabetes 2015;6(8):1073.

81. Chon JY, Moon HS. Salivary cortisol concentration changes after epidural steroid injection. Pain Physician 2012;15(6):461–6.

82. Jacobs S, Pullan PT, Potter JM, et al. Adrenal suppression following extradural steroids. Anaesthesia 1983;38(10):953–6.

83. Bayman E, Drake AJ. Adrenal suppression with glucocorticoid therapy: still a problem after all these years? Arch Dis Child 2017;102(4):338–9.

84. Kim S, Hwang B. Relationship between bone mineral density and the frequent administration of epidural steroid injections in postmenopausal women with low back pain. Pain Res Manag 2014;19(1):30–4.

85. Dubois EF, Wagemans MF, Verdouw BC, et al. Lack of relationships between cumulative methylprednisolone dose and bone mineral density in healthy men and postmenopausal women with chronic low back pain. Clin Rheumatol 2003;22(1):12–7.

86. Maillefert JF, Aho S, Huguenin MC, et al. Systemic effects of epidural dexamethasone injections. Rev Rhum Engl Ed 1995;62(6):429–32.

87. Danielson KD, Harrast MA. Focal spinal epidural lipomatosis after a single epidural steroid injection. PM&R 2011;3(6):590–3.

88. Gitkind AI, Shah B, Thomas M. Epidural corticosteroid injections as a possible cause of menorrhagia: a case report. Pain Med 2010;11(5):713–5.

89. Kim EC, Kim MS. Acute bilateral retinal hemorrhages and unilateral sixth cranial nerve palsy after inadvertent epidural anaesthetic injection and subsequent dural puncture. Can J Ophthalmol 2010;45(5):542–3.

90. Suh-Burgmann E, Hung Y-Y, Mura J. Abnormal vaginal bleeding after epidural steroid injection: a paired observation cohort study. Am J Obstet Gynecol 2013;209(3):206.e1-6.

91. Tuel SM, Meythaler JM, Cross LL. Cushing's syndrome from epidural methylprednisolone. Pain 1990;40(1):81–4.

92. Dietrich TJ, Sutter R, Froehlich JM, et al. Particulate versus non-particulate steroids for lumbar transforaminal or interlaminar epidural steroid injections: an update. Skeletal Radiol 2015;44(2):149–55.

93. O'Donnell CJ, Cano WG. Allergic reactions to gadodiamide following interventional spinal procedures: a report of 4 cases. Arch Phys Med Rehabil 2007; 88(11):1465–7.

94. American College of Radiolofy Manual on Contrast Media V10.2. 2016. Available at: https://www.acr.org/Quality-Safety/Resources/Contrast-Manual. Accessed July 11, 207.

95. Schopp JG, Iyer RS, Wang CL, et al. Allergic reactions to iodinated contrast media: premedication considerations for patients at risk. Emerg Radiol 2013;20(4): 299–306.

96. Safriel Y, Ali M, Hayt M, et al. Gadolinium use in spine procedures for patients with allergy to iodinated contrast: experience of 127 procedures. AJNR Am J Neuroradiol 2006;27(6):1194–7.

97. Li A, Wong CS, Wong MK, et al. Acute adverse reactions to magnetic resonance contrast media: gadolinium chelates. Br J Radiol 2006;79(941):368–71.

Sacroiliac Joint Interventions

David A. Soto Quijano, MD*, Eduardo Otero Loperena, MD

KEYWORDS

- Sacroiliac joint • Sacroilitis • Sacroiliac joint injections • Sacral lateral branch block
- Sacral lateral branch radiofrequency ablation

KEY POINTS

- Sacroiliac joint (SIJ) pain is an important cause of lower back problems.
- Multiple SIJ injection techniques have been proposed over the years to help in the diagnosis and treatment of this condition.
- SIJ innervation is complex and variable, and truly intra-articular injections are sometimes difficult to obtain.
- Intraarticular injections, periarticular injections, sacral branch blocks and radiofrequency ablation, both fluoroscopy guided and ultrasound guided, have been used to provide relief for patient with SIJ pain.
- Prolotherapy, platelet rich plasma injections and botulism toxin injections are also performed in the sacroiliac joint.

ANATOMY

The sacroiliac joint (SIJ) is the largest axial joint in the body. It consists of the articulation of the lateral sacrum with the posteromedial ilium and is considered part synovial and part syndesmosis. Together with the symphysis pubis joint, it transfers weight from the spine to the lower limb and provides certain elasticity to the pelvic ring.[1]

The SIJ stability is provided by several strong ligaments: the long and short posterior sacroiliac, the anterior sacroiliac, the sacrotuberous, the sacrospinous, and the iliolumbar ligaments. The posterior interosseous ligament forms the syndesmosis and the posterior border of the joint because there is no posterior joint capsule. SIJs have no muscles that control their movements directly, but their stability and motion are influenced by many muscles that directly control lumbar back, hip joints, and pelvis. The SIJs have limited mobility, but allow up to 4° of rotation and 1.6 mm of gliding. With age, the articular surfaces of the SIJs become more irregular, restricting movement and adding strength to the joint.[1]

The author has nothing to disclose.
Physical Medicine and Rehabilitation Residency Program, VA Caribbean Healthcare System, 10 Casia Street, San Juan, PR 00921, USA
* Corresponding author.
E-mail address: David.soto-quijano@va.gov

Phys Med Rehabil Clin N Am 29 (2018) 171–183
https://doi.org/10.1016/j.pmr.2017.09.004
pmr.theclinics.com

The posterior SIJ sensory innervation is provided by dorsal rami from S1-S3 via lateral branches and L4-L5 via medial branches. Anteriorly, the joint sensory innervation is provided by lumbosacral plexus through the lateral branches of posterior primary rami from L2 to S2. Contributions from superior gluteal and obturator nerves and other anatomic variations are also reported.[1,2]

Physical Examination

Specific tests for SIJ pain are divided into motion tests and provocation tests. Their reliability is operator dependent[3] and usually low.[4] Studies have reported that, in any patient, the diagnosis of SIJ pain has a sensitivity of 94% and a specificity of 78% when a patient presents positive responses to at least 3 of the following examination maneuvers: FABER, thigh trust, Gaenslen, distraction, sacral thrust, and compression test.[5,6] The use of provocative tests before and after injections to assess effectiveness is also controversial.[7]

Diagnostic Tests

In cases of sacroiliitis associated with spondyloarthropathies or traumatic disruption of joint, plain radiographs, MRI, and radionuclide bone scanning can identify characteristic changes, such as sclerosis, erosions, or ankylosis. However, in the absence of these diagnoses, the correlation of radiographic findings and patient pain is poor.[5]

Diagnostic blocks are also debated. Target-specificity is essential for a local anesthetic injection to be valid and the SIJ innervation is complex and variable. In addition, truly intra-articular injections are sometimes difficult to obtain. Periarticular injection can miss the innervation, and intra-articular SIJ diagnostic block may miss painful periarticular structures, making the interpretation of the injection inaccurate and its predictive value regarding response to further treatment, including other injections, radiofrequency ablation (RFA), neurostimulation, and/or SIJ surgical fusion, unreliable.[5,8]

Another gray area is the percent of pain alleviation after a block necessary to consider the test positive. High-quality studies about the diagnostic accuracy of sacroiliac intra-articular injections considered a relief of at least 70% to 75% as a positive result.[9] In the interventional pain practice policies published by the American Society of Interventional Pain Physicians, pain relief of 75% is used to consider a SIJ diagnostic injection as positive.[10] However, the International Society for the Advancement of Spinal Surgery criteria to consider minimally invasive SIJ fusion used a decrease in pain of >50% after a fluoroscopically guided diagnostic intra-articular SIJ block as a confirmation of SIJ as a pain generator.[11]

As in any other procedure, unexpected complications can arise after an SIJ injection. In a retrospective study, vasovagal reactions were the most common immediate adverse event, whereas injection-site soreness, pain exacerbation, and facial flushing and/or sweating were reported days later.[12] Other less common complications that have been described include herpes simplex and gas gangrene.[13,14]

SACROILIAC JOINT INTERVENTIONS
Periarticular Sacroiliac Fluoroscopic-Guided Injections

The patient is placed prone, and injection site is identified by obtaining a 15° to 20° oblique fluoroscopic view and aligning the medial edge of the posterior superior iliac spine (PSIS) with the medial edge of the SIJ line. A 22-g 3.5- to 5-inch-long spinal needle with curved tip is advanced in line with fluoroscopic beam targeting the point immediately medial and inferior to PSIS, making contact with the interosseous ligaments. Once there, the needle is rotated medially and advanced to the sacrum. Contrast medium is injected and expected to spread medial to SIJ in both caudal and cranial directions. Two milliliters of combined anesthetic and corticosteroid is then injected.[15] Nacey and colleagues[16] reviewed the records of 113 fluoroscopically guided SIJ injections with of 0.5 mL of bupivacaine and 0.5 mL (20 mg) of triamcinolone. Two musculoskeletal radiologists determined that 55 procedures were intra-articular and 58 were periarticular. Preinjection, immediate, and 1-week postinjection pain scores (0–10 numeric rating scale [NRS]) were found with no significant difference in the pain relief with intra-articular versus periarticular injections.

A retrospective review of 2 large case series compared patient responses to SIJ intra-articular injections versus combined intra-articular and periarticular injection of anesthetic and corticosteroids. The combined group showed a significantly higher percent of patients with greater than 50% of pain relief at 3-month follow-up.[15]

Intra-articular Sacroiliac Injection

Fluoroscopy-guided intra-articular sacroiliac joint injection
Multiple fluoroscopy-guided SIJ injection techniques have been proposed over the years probably because of the highly variable and complex SIJ anatomy and the difficulty identifying the posterior articular line.

Classic Hendrix technique With the technique of Hendrix and colleagues,[17] the patient is in the prone position, and an initial anteroposterior (AP) view with caudocranial angulation of fluoroscopy tube is taken. Then, the fluoroscope is adjusted medially or laterally by 5° until the inferior anterior and posterior joint spaces overlap. The inferior articular border is then marked for needle entry, and a 22-g 3.5-inch-long needle is then inserted vertically in-plane with the fluoroscope. After each 3 mm that the needle is advanced, its position should be checked fluoroscopically. About 3 to 5 cm from the skin surface, the depth of the needle penetration should be checked with a full lateral view. Then, with the AP view, the intra-articular position is confirmed with injection of 0.5 to 1.5 mL of contrast, which will be seen flowing superiorly if placed correctly.[18]

This technique is the most used intra-articular steroid SIJ injection technique. Although it is generally accepted as effective, a meta-analysis of SIJ interventions concluded that there is a lack of good studies to prove its effect. The evidence is limited to Level III or IV.[9]

Sacroiliac joint approach with only fluoroscopic anteroposterior view Khuba and colleagues[19] showed that in the initial true AP view, 70% of patients will show 2 SIJ spaces, with the medial joint space representing the posterior, and the lateral space representing the anterior SIJ. They proposed that the injection can be done with only initial unadjusted AP view, inserting a 22-g 3.5-inch-long needle on a posterior approach directed in-plane with fluoroscope toward the inferior third of the medial joint space. The tip of the needle should be slightly bent to guide the needle in the oblique direction of the joint once entered. In 30% of the patients in which the SIJ was seen as a straight line rather than 2 joint spaces in the AP view, the image intensifier of the fluoroscope was tilted cranially to elongate the image of the lower part of the posterior SIJ. The same 22-g 3.5-inch-long needle is then inserted in its distal 1 cm. Needle position was confirmed by injecting 0.3 to 0.5 of radiopaque contrast medium and had optimal contrast flow in 93% of patients. This technique has the advantage of fewer fluoroscopic views, less procedure time, and decreased radiation exposure. To the authors' knowledge, there are no studies published comparing the efficacy of this technique versus other SIJ injection techniques.

Lateral view technique Kasliwal and Sapana[20] proposed a modified Hendrix technique in which the lateral view is more important to confirm an adequate placement. The patient is placed prone and, as in Hendrix technique, the C-arm is angled until the silhouettes of the posterior and the anterior aspects of the SIJ overlap. A 3.5-inch-long needle is directed toward the lower third of the SIJ. With ipsilateral and contralateral oblique views, the needle is confirmed to be between the joint lines in the joint space and not on the bone. Then, the lateral view of fluoroscopy is used to guide the needle tip and to keep it at or above the S2 foramen ventral opening in the anterior one-third of the SIJ. Once the needle is in place, the contrast is injected and expected to travel cephalad in a flask-shaped manner. The investigators reported an accuracy of 93% of intra-articular needle placement, and relief of greater than 50% of pain in 96% of the patients (N = 30) injected with this technique.

The double needle technique Gupta[21] described another technique for difficult SIJ injections. First, a 3.5-inch-long needle is advanced toward the lower third of the SIJ following the Hendrix technique. Then, its position is checked with dynamic fluoroscopy in the right and left directions. If needle tip appears out of the joint and into the bone, a second needle is advanced to newly identified SIJ line and checked with dynamic fluoroscopy before using contrast dye. Once both needles are in place, dye is injected in the needle most likely to be inside the joint. If the contrast pattern is not satisfactory, then contrast is injected in the other needle. The author reported an increase in intra-articular needle placement accuracy in difficult patients when using this technique. To the author's knowledge, there are no studies evaluating the efficacy of this technique.

The upper one-third joint technique Park and colleagues[22] published an SIJ injection technique that can be used in patients in which the joint space at the lower third of the joint is too narrow or covered with osteophytes. The patient is positioned prone, and anesthetic is infiltrated with lidocaine in the midline of L5-S1 interspinous space. Then, a 22-g 10-cm-long spinal needle is advanced directly to upper third of SIJ at a 45° angle. As the needle tip hits firm tissue on the silhouette of the iliac crest, the curved needle is rotated and advanced beyond the iliac crest line until a pop sensation is felt. Intra-articular placement is then confirmed with 0.2 to 0.5 mL of contrast injection and its spreading in a cephalocaudal direction. The author used this technique in 20 patients who had unsuccessful sacroiliac intra-articular injections using the lower one-third joint technique. Of the 20 patients, 18 (90%) reported improvement.

The combined intra-articular upper third joint and periarticular injection The patient is placed in the prone position as usual with the C-arm fluoroscopy in a 40 to 50 contralateral oblique view. Using a superior approach, a 26-g, 90-mm-long spinal needle is advanced laterally and caudally to the wedge shape formed by the medial border of the ilium and the lateral border of the sacral ala, aiming at the upper third of the SIJ, avoiding the PSIS. After obtaining an AP projection, the needle is further advanced laterally and caudally until its tip felt entered the joint. Contrast is used to confirm intra-articular access, and then 0.5 mL of 2% lidocaine and 10 mg triamcinolone acetonide (total volume 1.5 mL) is injected. The periarticular injection is performed using the same needle after completing the intra-articular injection. The needle is withdrawn cranially, and its periarticular placement is confirmed by injecting 0.5 mL of contrast material. Then, 0.3 mL of 2% lidocaine and 5 mg triamcinolone acetonide (total volume 1.5 mL) are injected. Do and colleagues[23] performed the procedure in 24 patients with persistent SIJ pain despite conservative management. The procedures obtained satisfactory arthrograms, and pain scores were significantly reduced at 2 weeks and 4 weeks after treatment, having a 79% reported satisfaction.

IMPORTANCE OF ARTHROGRAM PATTERN

A study of 54 subjects who underwent therapeutic SIJ corticosteroid injection focused on the relationship between the short-term efficacy and the arthrographic contrast patterns. They concluded that injections in which the contrast flow showed a cephalad extension of contrast dispersion outlining the superior aspect of the SIJ have a greater pain reduction at 2 weeks, when compared with those whose contrast flow showed poor cephalad extension of contrast that fails to reach the most superior portion of the joint. Both groups reported same relief at 8 weeks.[24]

Ultrasound-guided Intra-articular Sacroiliac Joint Injection

The patient is positioned prone, and the SIJ is visualized with a low-frequency (4-6 mHz) curvilinear probe in transverse position over the lower sacrum to identify the sacral hiatus. After identifying the sacral cornu, the probe is moved laterally until the lateral edge of the sacrum is observed and then cephalad until the bony contour of the medial border of the ileum is visualized. The cleft between the lateral sacral border and medial ileum border represents the posterior aspect of the SIJ. The probe then should be tilted in a caudal direction to identify the lower third of the SIJ.[25]

Another ultrasound approach for identifying structures and injection site is done by placing the transducer transverse over the PSIS and moving caudally until the SIJ cleft is visualized between the lateral border of sacrum and medial border of ileum. Moving caudally, the S1 and S2 neural foramina can be identified medially to the SIJ cleft in the upper SIJ. The lower third of the SIJ becomes evident by the flat contour of the iliac crest and the presence of the S2 foramen, which is localized 2 to 3 cm above the caudal pole of SIJ. Color Doppler is used to determine the presence of vascular structures.[26]

Once injection site is identified with either of the approaches mentioned above, the injections can be done with needle in-plane or out-of-plane of the transducer. With the in-plane approach, a 22-g 3.5-inch-long spinal needle is advanced in a medial to lateral direction toward the wedge-shaped SIJ joint cleft. After needle aspiration to rule out intravascular position, the injection can proceed. Visible spread of injectate outside the joint requires reposition of needle, until the injectate is confined to the joint. To perform the out-of-plane technique, the needle is inserted in a caudal-to-cephalad direction. Once the needle is in place, color Doppler can be used to visualize potential retrograde flow. Intravascular injection would be difficult to detect once the needle tip is deep into the joint capsule.

Ultrasound Guided Versus Fluoroscopy Guided

A study performed by Soneji and colleagues[26] compared fluoroscopy versus ultrasound-guided SI injections in 40 patients. They found no significant difference in pain scores after 1 month and after 3 months in patients who received fluoroscopy-guided versus those who received ultrasound-guided injections. They also reported similar functional outcomes and intra-articular injection rates. Jee and colleagues[27] published a similar study comparing the efficacy of ultrasound-guided versus fluoroscopy-guided SIJ intra-articular injections in 120 patients with non-inflammatory SIJ dysfunction. Although the fluoroscopy-guided SIJ approach exhibited a greater accuracy than the ultrasound-guided approach (98.2% vs 87.3%), function and pain relief improved in both groups without significant differences. Another study used 17 cadavers to test the reliability of ultrasound-guided SIJ injections. They confirmed with dissection that 88.2% of the injections were correctly placed inside the joints.[28]

Sacral Branches Block

Although the innervation of SIJ is complex and variable, nerve blocks have been used as diagnostic tools, and respondents have been considered for RFA of lateral sacral branches.[29]

Fluoroscopic guidance

For the 17-injection technique for sacral lateral branches block, the patient is placed in the usual prone position, and posteroanterior imaging through the L5-S1 disc space is obtained. For sacral lateral branch injections, needles are placed 8- to 10-mm peripheral to the posterior sacral foramina, using clock-face coordinates, with the center of the clock at the lateral margin of the foramen. At the S1 and S2 levels, on the right, needles are placed at the 2:30, 4:00, and 5:30 positions, and on the left, they are placed at the 9:30, 8:00, and 6:30 positions. At the S3 level, on the right, needles are placed at the 2:30 and 4:00 positions, and on the left, at the 9:30 and 8:00 positions. A standardized skin ruler is used to assure that the target needles are placed 8 to 10 mm from the lateral margin of the posterior sacral foramen at each segmental level. For these lateral branch injections, a minimal amount of contrast medium is initially injected under posteroanterior imaging to avoid epidural or venous flow and redirect the needle as needed. Then 0.2 mL of bupivacaine is injected. The needle is then pulled back approximately one bevel length (approximately 3 mm) and another 0.2 mL of the allocated agent is injected. The same protocol was followed at each target segment.

Dreyfuss and colleagues[30] performed a randomized controlled trial with 20 patients with SIJ pain. In 10 patients, they performed this technique and in 10 patients saline was injected as placebo. There was a significant decrease in pain in 7 of the patients in the active group and only on one in the placebo group.

Ultrasound guidance

For the ultrasound-guided lateral sacral branch block technique, the patient is placed in the prone position and the sacrum is scanned on the transverse plane. The caudal aspect of SIJ is located at or slightly above the S2 posterior foramen, and the posterior sacral foramina S1, S2, S3 are identified in the transverse plane moving the probe in a cephalad direction from the sacral cornu. The overlying cutaneous area is infiltrated with 0.3 mL of 2% lidocaine. The first block needle is positioned in a cephalad direction to the lateral crest in the midpoint between S2 and S3 using an in-plane technique, in a medial to lateral direction. The needle is confirmed in position with a sagittal view of sacrum with the 3 sacral foramina visualized in the same view. Then, 1.5 mL of 2% lidocaine is injected. The second block needle is inserted toward the lateral crest just above the S2, and the third needle block is directed to the lateral crest at the level of S1 posterior sacral foramina. In both points, 0.5 mL of 2% lidocaine is injected.[29]

Ultrasound Versus Fluoroscopic Guided Sacral Lateral Branches Blocks

In 2017, Finlayson and colleagues[29] published a randomized controlled trial comparing ultrasound- and fluoroscopy-guided sacral lateral branch blocks in 40 patients with chronic lower back pain. They used the 17-injection technique, and the ultrasound-guided technique described above. They concluded that the pain relief effect was similar in both groups 30 days after the procedures. However, the ultrasound technique required shorter performance time, required fewer needle passes, provided improved visibility at the S3 level, and caused less patient discomfort, less radiation exposure, and lower risk of vascular breach.

Radiofrequency Ablation

Intra-articular radiofrequency ablation

The intra-articular SIJ RFA, especially the pulsed radiofrequency (PRF), has been used with apparent success, but still needs more clinical trials to confirm their efficacy.[31] A case report of a 42-year-old patient with SIJ pain reported improvement after receiving intra-articular PRF with a pulse width of 10 ms, at 2 Hz, and 65 V for 10 minutes. The patient noted marked improvement of his pain: at 12-week follow-up, he was pain free, and at 6-month follow-up, there was mild pain over the SI region (NRS score 3).[32] However, a retrospective study of 20 patients who received intra-articular PRF stimulation of the SIJ for chronic SIJ pain that had not responded to intra-articular corticosteroid injection showed limited results. The NRS scores at 1, 2, and 3 months after PRF were significantly lower than those before PRF. Only 4 of the 20 patients (20%) reported successful pain relief (pain relief of ≥50%) and were satisfied with the PRF stimulation at 3 months after treatment. Intra-articular PRF stimulation of the SIJ was not successful in most patients (80% of all patients).[33]

Ferrante[34] described a series of 50 SIJ denervations using a leapfrog technique. The fluoroscopy view and needle approach are similar to the technique used for intra-articular SIJ injections. Anesthesia is obtained by local infiltration of lidocaine. The first radiofrequency (RF) probe is directed toward the inferior joint margin. A second probe is inserted more cephalad in the joint line within a distance less than 1 cm from the first probe to create a bipolar system. A third probe is placed 1 cm more cephalad to the second. Because of a lack of important motor nerves in the area, the sensory and motor prestimulation is not recommended for this procedure. The intra-articular location of each probe is confirmed by injection of contrast material on lateral and AP views. This technique creates a strip lesion of the posterior SIJ. The criteria for successful RF denervation were at least a 50% decrease in visual analogue score (VAS) for a period of at least 6 months; 36.4% of patients (12 of 33) met these criteria. The average duration of pain relief for those who responded was 12.0 ± 1.2 months.

Lateral branches radiofrequency ablation

a. The strip lesion technique results in L5 dorsal ramus and lateral dorsal S1-S3 periforaminal strip RFA. With the patient lying prone, local anesthesia is infiltrated over the S1, S2, and S3 foramina. Then a 20-g, 10-cm-long, 10-mm exposed curved tip cannula is inserted perpendicular to the skin down to the bone. The L5 posterior ramus is lesioned at the junction of the sacral ala and the root of the superior articular process of S1. On the right side, on each sacral foramina, a bipolar string lesion is made by placing needle tips between the 12 o'clock and 2 o'clock positions, after which the 12 o'clock needle is removed and placed at the 4 o'clock position where another lesion is made. Then, the 2 o'clock position needle is removed and placed at the 6 o'clock position for a last lesion. On the left side, the lesions are made in the same fashion but at 12 to 10 o'clock, 10 to 8 o'clock, and 8 to 6 o'clock positions. If the sacral foramen is large, more lesions are needed to cover the lateral hemicircle of the foramen but maintaining the interprobe positions within 5- to 6-mm distance. Burnham and colleagues[35] described this technique in 9 patients with excellent pain relief and satisfaction scores after 12-month follow-up in 8 out of 9 patients.

b. Bellini and Barbieri[36] used a single multielectrode RF probe positioned through a single percutaneous entry point along the sacrum, lateral to the sacral foramina and medial to the SIJ. One hundred two treatments were reported; 91.8% resulted in a reduction of more than 50% pain intensity relief at 1 month, 81.6% at 3 months, 59.16% at 6 months, and 35.7% at 1 year.

c. The 3-puncture technique targets the lateral sacral branches S1-S3 and uses a unipolar lesion. The patient is placed prone; the S1 dorsal foramen is identified, and the fluoroscope is accommodated until the foramen is in "tunnel vision view." After sterilization and anesthesia, an RF cannula is inserted to the bone over the lateral upper quadrant of the S1 dorsal foramen. The cannula tip should be place alongside the nerve. Next, a lateral view is taken to confirm position and avoid placing the needle too close to the ventral foramen. Then, the fluoroscope is moved caudally for better visualization of the S2 and S3 foramina, and the procedure described above is repeated at those levels. The needles should be forming a straight line. Then, the needle stylet in the cannula is replaced by the thermistor electrodes, and sensory and motor prestimulation is done to confirm position. No muscle contraction should be felt by patient or physician in the urogenital or anal region. Then, the lesions are made on each of the sacral levels. Buijs and colleagues[37] described this procedure in 43 patients, and at 12-week follow-up, 34.9% referred complete pain relief, and 32.6% referred relief of greater than 50%. No complications were described.

d. A similar procedure was described by Biswas and colleagues[38] with water-cooled RF. With this procedure, the patient is placed in the prone position, and skin overlying each SIJ area is infiltrated with 1% lidocaine after sterile preparation of the site. With fluoroscopy guidance, three 27-g 3.5-inch-long Quincke needles are placed into S1 through S3 posterior sacral foramina to establish internal reference points for RF probe placement. Beginning at the S1 level, an RF probe introducer with stylet is inserted on the bone of the posterior sacrum, lying at a safe distance from the sacral foramina as guided by internal reference points and an epsilon marker. RF probe is subsequently inserted through the same introducer and placement is confirmed in the lateral view. Tissue impedance, motor testing, and sensory testing are done to corroborate correct probe placement. Following instillation of 0.25% bupivacaine 1 mL for each lesion area, WC-RF (water-cooled radiofrequency) energy is delivered for 150 seconds with 60°C as the target electrode temperature. Two or 3 lesions are created at each sacral level about 1 cm apart from one another using an epsilon ruler, from S1 to S3 on both sides.

e. The guide-block technique is used to perform the ablation of the lateral branches of the S1, S2, and S3 dorsal rami as well as the L5 dorsal ramus by creating a continuous strip lesion along a straight line lateral to the sacral foramen. Seven to 9 RF needles are placed perpendicular to the surface plane of the sacrum parallel to each other with a distance of 10 mm between each pair of adjacent needles. The RF probes must be precisely parallel to each other in order to perform bipolar RFA in a continuous strip lesion. This procedure is technically challenging and time consuming, so a guide block 90 mm long, 10 mm wide, and 6 mm thick with 9 through-holes 10 mm apart along a straight line is used. The diameter of the through-holes allows a 20-g, straight RF needle to pass through easily without waggling.

With this technique, the patient is placed in the prone position as usual, and the skin is prepared and draped with sterile technique. The guide block is placed on the skin on the side affected over the sacrum and aligned under fluoroscopy so that the cranial radiopaque marker is on top of the sacral ala, just lateral to the base of the S1 superior articular process of the L5-S1 facet joint and the most caudal one lateral and distal to the lateral border of the S3 foramen. The location of the guide block is marked with a marking pen, and the guide block is removed to expose the skin underneath. Then, after local anesthesia is obtained with lidocaine, the guide block is then loaded with 7 RF needles, with the tips of the needles barely passing through the through-holes and returned to its original position. The needles are then advanced about 10 mm into the skin, one at a time. Once all of the needles are advanced to the dorsal surface of the sacrum until bone contact, a fluoroscopy lateral view confirms that none of the needles went into the sacral foramen or landed on the posterior iliac crests. The stylets of the needles are then removed; 2 mL of 1% lidocaine is injected through each needle, and a strip lesion is created by delivering RF energy (85°C for 150 seconds) through 4 electrodes, making 2 controlled lesions along the strip at a time. Three sequential lesions were made by the combinations of needle connections. Upon completion of the procedure, all the needles are removed. This technique was shown to decrease operating time by 50% compared with a regular pulsed RFA procedure, decreased radiograph exposure by 80%, and higher percent of patients with achieved persistent 50% or more pain relief after 12 months of follow-up.[39]

Effectiveness of RFA

A prospective, randomized, and experimental study evaluated 60 patients with SIJ pain for more than 3 months. Patients were randomized into a group that received 2 intra-articular sacroiliac injections of local anesthetic/corticosteroid guided by ultrasound in 7 days, a group that received conventional bipolar RF over the lateral branch nerves of S1, S2, and S3 with a distance between needles of 1 cm and a third group who received bipolar RF with a needle distance of more than 1 cm. At 1 month, pain reduction was greater than 50% in the 3 groups. However, at 3 and 12 months, the groups that received radioablation reported improvement of the pain, whereas the patients who received intra-articular injections did not have a significant reduction in pain.[40]

A meta-analysis of the effectiveness of RFA on the treatment of SIJ pain evaluated 10 articles. The main outcome measure was a reduction of pain by $\geq$50% 6 and 3 months after RFA procedure. The investigators concluded that RFA is an effective treatment of SIJ pain at 3 months and 6 months, but the conclusions are limited by the available literature and lack of randomized controlled trials.[41]

A systematic review of therapeutic effectiveness of all SIJ interventions, including intra-articular injections, periarticular injections, conventional RF, and cooled RF neurotomy, reported that greatest evidence supports the cooled RF neurotomy of lateral branches based on 2 randomized controlled trials and 2 observational studies. The other interventions have weaker evidence to support them.[9]

Prolotherapy

Prolotherapy is the injection of irritant solution, usually hyperosmolar dextrose, into a joint space, ligament, or tendon insertion to attract inflammatory mediators, stimulate the release of growth factors, and induce tissue repair. It has been used for SIJ pain in periarticular and intra-articular areas to treat pain and sacral ligaments laxity. There is literature that supports that intra-articular sacroiliac prolotherapy with hyperosmolar dextrose provides longer lasting pain relief compared with steroid and anesthetic combination. However, more evidence is needed to determine its real effect, clinical indications, and the appropriate protocols.[42] A randomized controlled trial with 48 patients comparing pain and disability scores after intra-articular SIJ prolotherapy or steroid injection with fluoroscopy guidance showed no difference at 2 weeks follow-up but statistically significant difference in pain relief at 15 months follow-up favoring the prolotherapy group.[43] A prospective descriptive study showed that 75% of 25 patients that received 3 injections of hypertonic dextrose solution into the dorsal interosseous ligament of the affected SIJ reported improvement.[44]

Platelet-rich plasma

Plasma rich in platelets (PRP) is injected to modulate the anti-inflammatory pathway and repair the process of damaged tissue by activating macrophages and inducing collagen proliferation, cellular differentiation, vasodilation, and vascularization in areas with poor vascularization or poor inherent healing potential.[45] It has become very popular, but good studies to determine its usefulness are still lacking.

In 2016, Navani and Gupta[45] published 10 cases of SIJ pain refractory to physical therapy and anti-inflammatory medications that received injections of 4 mm of autologous PRP into the joint under fluoroscopic guidance. All the patients reported greater than 50% of pain relief at 12 months follow-up, and none reported complications, had hospital visits, or received another kind of additional therapy. A randomized controlled study compared intra-articular steroid versus PRP ultrasound-guided injections in 40 patients. At 4 weeks, the pain relief and disability scores in both groups were similar, but at 3 months, the pain and functional improvement persisted in the PRP group and deteriorated in the steroid group.[46] A case series described patients whose improvement was maintained 4 years after an ultrasound-guided PRP injection for SIJ dysfunction.[47]

Botulinum toxin

Initially, the pain relief that resulted after using botulinum toxin was attributed to reduction of muscle overactivity in patients with dystonia and headaches. Then, when the same pain relief was observed in other nonmuscular tissues, such as intra-articular space, other mechanisms were proposed. Botulinum toxin might reduce local release of nociceptive neuropeptides, which would also inhibit neurogenic inflammation.[48] It also could lead to reduction of central sensitization to pain by controlling sensory input into and autonomic output from spinal cord neurons and may stimulate the release of naturally secreted analgesics, such as enkephalins.[48]

A prospective case control study was published in 2010 by Lee and colleagues[48] comparing the clinical effectiveness of fluoroscopy-guided periarticular botulinum toxin SIJ injections with fluoroscopy-guided periarticular steroid and anesthetic combination in patients with SIJ pain. They found that the pain control was similar on evaluation 1 month after the procedure, but persisted in the botulinum toxin group with high statistical significance at 2 and 3 months follow-up.

REFERENCES

1. Magee DJ. "Pelvis." Orthopedic physical assessment. 6th edition. St Louis (MO): Elsevier Saunders; 2014. p. 649–88.
2. Cox RC, Fortin JD. The anatomy of the lateral branches of the sacral dorsal rami: implications for radiofrequency ablation. Pain Physician 2014;17(5):459–64.
3. Cusi MF. Paradigm for assessment and treatment of SIJ mechanical dysfunction. J Bodyw Mov Ther 2010;14(2):152–61.
4. Slipman CW, Sterenfeld EB, Chou LH, et al. The predictive value of provocative sacroiliac joint stress maneuvers in the diagnosis of sacroiliac joint syndrome. Arch Phys Med Rehabil 1998;79(3):288–92.
5. Kennedy DJ, Engel A, Kreiner DS, et al. Fluoroscopically guided diagnostic and therapeutic intra-articular sacroiliac joint injections: a systematic review. Pain Med 2015;16(8):1500–18.
6. Laslett M, Aprill CN, Mcdonald B, et al. Diagnosis of sacroiliac joint pain: validity of individual provocation tests and composites of tests. Man Ther 2005;10: 207–18.
7. Stanford G, Burnham RS. Is it useful to repeat sacroiliac joint provocative tests post-block? Pain Med 2010;11(12):1774–6.

8. Polly D, Cher D, Whang PG, et al, INSITE Study Group. Does level of response to SI joint block predict response to SI joint fusion? Int J Spine Surg 2016;10:4.

9. Simopoulos TT, Manchikanti L, Gupta S. Systematic review of the diagnostic accuracy and therapeutic effectiveness of sacroiliac joint interventions. Pain Physician 2015;18:E713–56.

10. Manchikanti L, Abdi S, Atluri S, et al. An update of comprehensive evidence based guidelines for interventional techniques in chronic spinal pain. Part II: guidance and recommendations. Pain Physician 2013;16(2 Suppl):S49–283.

11. Lorio MP. ISASS policy 2016 update: minimally invasive sacroiliac joint fusion. Int J Spine Surg 2016;10:26.

12. Plastaras CT, Joshi AB, Garvan C, et al. Adverse events associated with fluoroscopically guided sacroiliac joint injections. PM R 2012;4(7):473–8.

13. Meydani A, Schwartz RA, Foye PM, et al. Herpes simplex following intra-articular sacroiliac corticosteroid injection. Acta Dermatovenerol Alp Pannonica Adriat 2009;18(3):135–7.

14. Kurnutala LN, Ghatol D, Upadhyay A. Clostridium sacroiliitis (gas gangrene) following sacroiliac joint injection–case report and review of the literature. Pain Physician 2015;18(4):E629–32.

15. Borowsky CD, Fagen G. Sources of sacroiliac region pain: insights gained from a study comparing standard intra-articular injection with a technique combining intra- and peri-articular injection. Arch Phys Med Rehabil 2008;89(11):2048–56.

16. Nacey NC, Patrie JT, Fox MG. Fluoroscopically guided sacroiliac joint injections: comparison of the effects of intraarticular and periarticular injections on immediate and short-term pain relief. AJR Am J Roentgenol 2016;207(5):1055–61.

17. Hendrix RW, Lin PJ, Kane WJ. Simplified aspiration or injection technique for the sacro-iliac joint. J Bone Joint Surg Am 1982;64(8):1249–52.

18. Liliang PC, Liang CL, Lu K, et al. Modified fluoroscopy-guided sacroiliac joint injection: a technical report. Pain Med 2014;15(9):1477–80.

19. Khuba S, Agarwal A, Gautam S, et al. Fluoroscopic sacroiliac joint injection: is oblique angulation really necessary. Pain Physician 2016;19:E1135–8.

20. Kasliwal PJ, Sapana K. Fluoroscopy-guided sacroiliac joint injection: description of a modified technique. Pain Physician 2016;19:E329–37.

21. Gupta S. Double needle technique: an alternative method for performing difficult sacroiliac joint injections. Pain Physician 2011;14(3):281–4.

22. Park J, Park HJ, Moon DE, et al. Radiologic analysis and clinical study of the upper one-thrid joint technique for fluoroscopically guided sacroiliac joint injection. Pain Physician 2015;18:495–503.

23. Do KH, Ahn SH, Jones R. A new sacroiliac joint injection technique and its short-term effect on chronic sacroiliac region pain. Pain Med 2016;17(10):1809–13.

24. Scholten PM, Patel SI, Christos PJ, et al. Short-term efficacy of sacroiliac joint corticosteroid injection based on arthrographic contrast patterns. PM R 2015;7(4):385–91.

25. Chang WH, Lew HL, Chen CP. Ultrasound-guided sacroiliac joint injection technique. Am J Phys Med Rehabil 2013;92(3):278–9.

26. Soneji N, Bhatia A, Seib R, et al. Comparison of fluoroscopy and ultrasound guidance for sacroiliac joint injection in patients with chronic low back pain. Pain Pract 2015;16(5):537–44.

27. Jee H, Lee JH, Park KD, et al. Ultrasound-guided versus fluoroscopy-guided sacroiliac joint intra-articular injections in the noninflammatory sacroiliac joint dysfunction: a prospective, randomized, single-blinded study. Arch Phys Med Rehabil 2014;95(2):330–7.

28. Perry JM, Colberg RE, Dault SL, et al. A cadaveric study assessing the accuracy of ultrasound-guided sacroiliac joint injections. PM R 2016;8(12):1168–72.
29. Finlayson RJ, Etheridge JP, Elgueta MF, et al. A randomized comparison between ultrasound- and fluoroscopy-guided sacral lateral branch blocks. Reg Anesth Pain Med 2017;42(3):400–6.
30. Dreyfuss P, Henning T, Malladi N, et al. The ability of multi-site, multi-depth sacral lateral branch blocks to anesthetize the sacroiliac joint complex. Pain Med 2009; 10(4):679–88.
31. Facchini G, Spinnato P, Guglielmi G, et al. A comprehensive review of pulsed radiofrequency in the treatment of pain associated with different spinal conditions. Br J Radiol 2017;90(1073):20150406.
32. Sluijter ME, Teixeira A, Serra V, et al. Intra-articular application of pulsed radiofrequency for arthrogenic pain—report of six cases. Pain Pract 2008;8(1):57–61.
33. Chang MC, Ahn SH. The effect of intra-articular stimulation by pulsed radiofrequency on chronic sacroiliac joint pain refractory to intra-articular corticosteroid injection: a retrospective study. Medicine (Baltimore) 2017;96(26):e7367.
34. Ferrante F. Radiofrequency sacroiliac joint denervation for sacroiliac syndrome. Reg Anesth Pain Med 2001;26(2):137–42.
35. Burnham R, Yasui Y. An alternate method of radiofrequency neurotomy of the sacroiliac joint: a pilot study of the effect on pain, function, and satisfaction. Reg Anesth Pain Med 2007;32(1):12–9.
36. Bellini M, Barbieri M. Single strip lesions radiofrequency denervation for treatment of sacroiliac joint pain: two years' results. Anaesthesiol Intensive Ther 2016;48(1):19–22.
37. Buijs EJ, Kamphuis ET, Groen GJ. Radiofrequency treatment of sacroiliac joint-related pain aimed at the first three sacral dorsal rami: a minimal approach. Pain Clin 2004;16(2):139–46.
38. Biswas B, Dey S, Biswas S, et al. Water-cooled radiofrequency neuroablation for sacroiliac joint dysfunctional pain. J Anaesthesiol Clin Pharmacol 2016;32(4):525.
39. Cheng J, Chen SL, Zimmerman N, et al. A new radiofrequency ablation procedure to treat sacroiliac joint pain. Pain Physician 2016;19:603–5.
40. Cánovas Martínez L, Orduña Valls J, Paramés Mosquera E, et al. Sacroiliac joint pain: prospective, randomised, experimental and comparative study of thermal radiofrequency with sacroiliac joint block. Rev Esp Anestesiol Reanim 2016; 63(5):267–72.
41. Aydin SM, Gharibo CG, Mehnert M, et al. The role of radiofrequency ablation for sacroiliac joint pain: a meta-analysis. PM R 2010;2(9):842–51.
42. Distel LM, Best TM. Prolotherapy: a clinical review of its role in treating chronic musculoskeletal pain. PM R 2011;3(6 Suppl 1):S78–81.
43. Kim WM, Hyung GL, Cheol WJ, et al. A randomized controlled trial of intra-articular prolotherapy versus steroid injection for sacroiliac joint pain. J Altern Complement Med 2010;16(12):1285–90.
44. Cusi M, Saunders J, Hungerford B, et al. The use of prolotherapy in the sacroiliac joint. Br J Sports Med 2010;44(2):100–4.
45. Navani A, Gupta D. Role of intra-articular platelet-rich plasma in sacroiliac joint pain. Tech Reg Anesth Pain Manag 2015;19(1–2):54–9.
46. Singla V, Batra YK, Bharti N, et al. Steroid vs. platelet-rich plasma in ultrasound-guided sacroiliac joint injection for chronic low back pain. Pain Pract 2017;17(6): 782–91.

47. Ko GD, Mindra S, Lawson GE, et al. Case series of ultrasound-guided platelet-rich plasma injections for sacroiliac joint dysfunction. J Back Musculoskelet Rehabil 2017;30(2):363–70.
48. Lee JH, Lee SH, Song SH. Clinical effectiveness of Botulinum Toxin A compared to a mixture of steroid and local anesthetics as a treatment for sacroiliac joint pain. Pain Med 2010;11(5):692–700.

Printed and bound by CPI Group (UK) Ltd, Croydon, CR0 4YY

07/10/2024

01040505-0020